FORMULARY OF
EQUINE MEDICINE

FORMULARY OF
EQUINE MEDICINE

COMPILED BY THE STAFF OF
The Division of Equine Studies
Department of Veterinary Clinical Science
University of Liverpool
Leahurst, Wirral, L64 7TE, UK

EDITED BY
D. C. KNOTTENBELT

LIVERPOOL UNIVERSITY PRESS

First published 1991 by the
Department of Veterinary Clinical Science,
University of Liverpool

Second edition published 1992 by
Liverpool University Press,
PO Box 147, Liverpool, L69 3BX

British Library Cataloguing-in-Publication Data
A British Library CIP Record is available
ISBN 0 85323 357 8

Printed in the European Community by
Page Bros, Norwich

CONTENTS

		PAGE
Vital Signs		1
Sample Collection Instructions		2
Normal values	a) Haematology	3
	b) Biochemical parameters	4
	c) Acid-Base Balance	5
	d) Enzymes	6
	e) Blood Coagulation	7
	f) Cerebro-spinal fluid	7
	g) Synovial Fluid	8
	h) Peritoneal / Pleural Fluid	8
	i) Urinalysis	9
Reproductive Data	a) Female	11
	b) Male	13
Diagnostic Tests	i) BSP Clearance	17
	ii) Glucose Absorbtion	17
	iii) Sodium Sulphanilate Clearance	18
	iv) Zinc Sulphate Turbidity Test	18
	v) Cryptorchidism	19
	vi) Paracentesis Abdominus	20
	vii) Paracentesis Thoracis	20
	viii) Transtracheal Wash	21
	ix) Bronchio-alveolar Lavage	21
	x) Bone Marrow Biopsy	22
	xi) Liver Biopsy	22
	xi) Renal Clearance ratios	23
	xii) Pituitary - Adrenal (ACTH) Tests	24
	xiii) Thyroid Stimulation Test	24
Electrocardiographic Data		27
Index of Drugs/Therapeutic Data		33
	Prescription abbreviations	34
	Drug Categorization	35
	1) Drugs Acting on CNS	37
	a) CNS/Respiratory stimulants	38
	b) Analgesics	39
	c) Tranquilisers and Sedative	42
	d) Anaesthetic Agents	44
	i) Volatile/Gases	44
	ii) Intravenous	45
	e) Anticonvulsants	47
	f) Muscle Relaxants	49
	g) Parasympathomimetics	50
	h) Parasympatholytics	50
	i) Sympathomimetics	51
	j) Sympatholytics	53
	k) Opiate Antagonists	54
	l) Euthenasia Solutions	55

2) Drugs Acting on Cardiovascular System   59
   a) Antiarrythmics   60
   b) Cardiac Glycosides   61
   c) Anticholinergics   61
   d) Vasodilators   62
   e) Shock Treatments   63
3) Drugs acting on Respiratory System   65
   a) Bronchodilators   67
   b) Antihistamines   69
   c) Antitussives   70
   d) Mucolytics   71

4) Drugs acting on Urinary System   73
   a) Diuretics   75

5) Drugs acting on Gastro-Intestinal System   79
   a) Antacids/Anti-ulcer   80
   b) Intestinal stimulants   81
   c) Intestinal sedatives/antispasmodics   81
   d) Laxatives/cathartics   82
   e) Antidiarrhoeals   84

6) Hormones   87
   a) Prostaglandins   88
   b) Sex/Trophic hormones   89
   c) Anabolic Steroids   92
   d) Posterior Pituitary   92
   e) Adrenal Corticoids   93
   f) Non steroidal antiinflamatories   96
   g) Others   99

7) Antiinfective Drugs   101
   a) Anthelmintics   103
   b) Antibiotics   108
   c) Sulphonamides   113
   d) Other antibacterials   114
   e) Antifungals   115
   f) Antiprotozoals   117
   g) Parasiticides   118

8) Blood Modifying Drugs   123
   a) Anti-coagulants   124
   b) Coagulants   126
   c) Haematinics   127
   d) Vitamins   128
   e) Electrolytes   131

9) Vaccines/Antisera   135

10) Miscellaneous Drugs   141
     a) Local anaesthetics   143
     b) Eye Preparations   144
         i) Antibiotics   144
         ii) Midriatics   145
         iii) Miotics   146
         iv) Anaesthetics   146
         v) Steroids   147
         vi) Artificial Tears   148
         vii) Diagnostic/Miscellaneous   149
     c) Skin Preparations   150
         i) Antiseptics/disinfectants   150
         ii)Parasiticides   150
         iii) Astringents   151
         iv) Poultices   151
         v) Casting Materials   152
     d) Joint preparations   153
     e) Antidotes/antitoxins   154
     f) Suture Materials   155
     Drugs contraindicated in the horse   156

Appendices: 161
Weight Estimation Methods   Appendix 1   162

Metric Conversion/Molecular Weights   Appendix 2   163

SI Conversion Factors   Appendix 3   164

Ageing of Horses (Dental)   Appendix 4   165

Humane Destruction of Horses   Appendix 5   173

Bandaging Techniques for Horses   Appendix 6   174

Diagnostic Nerve Block Sites   Appendix 6   177

Neonatal Assessment/SEPSIS SCORING   Appendix 7   181

Notifiable Diseases   Appendix 8   183

Investigative Protocols   Appendix 9   184
     Purchase examination   184
     Colic   185
     Lameness   186

Equipment for Equine Practice   187
     First Aid for Events/Racing etc   187
     Practice Car Boot List   188
Useful Addresses   Appendix 10   190
Index   193

Preface:

The formulary lists some haematological, biochemical, physiological and therapeutic data and is produced with the Final Year veterinary student and recent graduate in mind. It is not intended to be a definitive 'bible' for those wishing to specialise in a particular aspect of equine medicine. Extra pages have been inserted at convenient points for personal additions and notes. We hope it will prove useful and informative and make an effective contribution to the teaching of equine medicine.

The values given for vital signs, haematology and clinical chemistry in the first section are in International Metric (SI) units unless otherwise stated and are values which are accepted as being normal, although individual commercial and private laboratories may quote different normal ranges. Whilst every precaution has been taken to ensure accuracy we do not accept any liability for errors or omissions.

Indications, dosages and adverse reactions given in this booklet are not intended to be fully comprehensive. The dosages are those recommended by the manufacturers in their data sheets and literature inserts and are based on clinical experience. All doses are in mg/kg body weight unless otherwise stated.

Trade names are included with the generic names but the list of these cannot be definitive, and the mention or exclusion of any particular commercial product is not a recommendation or otherwise as to its value. Formulations of drugs are being released and withdrawn every year and this makes defintitive lists very difficult to construct. **Veterinary surgeons using this publication are warned that not all the drugs listed here are licensed for equine use and that appropriate considerations must be made for all such drugs before they are used.** The intention of this book is to identify the drugs and their uses and to leave the selection of drugs to the veterinarian concerned. Accordingly the drugs are not listed as "licensed" or "not-licensed" for equine use. It should be realised that new drugs are constantly being marketed and some are being removed from registration. Due note should be taken of the current status of individual products.

Acknowledgements:

The contributions of the staff of the Equine Division and Veterinary Anaesthesia are gratefully acknowledged. Particular thanks for their assistance are due to Professor Barrie Edwards, Drs John Cox and Stephen May, Mrs Luise Harrison, Ms Lesley Young and Ms Anne Gregg, and Messrs Chris Proudman and Chris Danton.

D.C.Knottenbelt BVM&S, DVM&S, MRCVS

NOTES

VITAL SIGNS, NORMAL VALUES AND DIAGNOSTIC TESTS

NORMAL VITAL SIGNS

	Pulse Rate (/min)	Respiration Rate (/min)	Temperature (Rectal) (°C)	Capillary Refill (secs)
Foal (newborn)	100-128	14-15	38.5-39.5	<2
Foal (7days)	80-120	14-16	38.0-39.0	<2
Foal (3months)	60-100	14-15	37.5-38.0	<2
Pony	45-55	12-15	37.5-38.0	<2
Thoroughbred	35-45	12-15	37.5-38.0	<2
Thoroughbred(fit)	25-40	10-15	37.5-38.5	<2

SAMPLE COLLECTION :

Note: The following are recommended by the Veterinary Pathology Laboratory at Leahurst.
Advisable to check anticoagulant requirements with laboratory before obtaining samples.
Consider effects of transport on samples, particularly when this involves postal services.

SAMPLES MARKED: * are BEST, + are ACCEPTABLE, 0 are UNACCEPTABLE

	EDTA (pink)	FlOx (grey)	Citrate (blue)	Li Hep (green)	Plain (red)			
Haematology	*	0	0	+	0	L	H	
Clotting Factors	0	0	*	0	0	L	H	
Glucose[12]	0	*	0	0	0			S
Phosphate	0	*	0	0	+		H	
Urea	+	0	+	+	*		H	
Total Prot[3]	0	0	+	+	*	L	H	
Albumin	0	0	+	+	*	L	H	
Globulin	0	0	0	+	*	L	H	
Fibrinogen	0	0	+	+	+			
Bilirubin	+	0	+	+	*		H	
Cholesterol	0	0	0	+	*			
Triglycerides	0	0	0	+	*	L		
Creatinine	0	0	0	+	*	L	H	
Lactate[4]	0	0	+	+	0			
Calcium	0	0	0	+	*			
Copper	0	0	0	+	*		H	
Sodium	0	0	0	0	*			
Chloride	0	0	0	0	*			
Blood gases	0	0	0	*	0	L	H	
Bicarbonate	0	0	0	*	0			
Ammonia	(special requirements for cooling etc check with Lab)							
Enzymes	0	0	0	+	*	L	H	S
Thyroid[5]	0	0	0	+	*			
Hormones[5]	0	0	0	*	*			S

H = affected by haemolysis, L = affected by lipaemia, S = serum separation should be immediate

---

[1] check sample - significant difference between blood/plasam/serum

[2] Separate plasma as soon as possible

[3] significant difference between serum and plasma

[4] Assay immediately

[5] Assay immediately (<2 hours)

NORMAL VALUES

NOTE: there are always critisisms of normal values in view of the individual variations within the population but the skilled clinician is invariably able to make critical judgements on their valididty.

A) Haematology :

Parameter(units)	Birth-3weeks	Pony/Mare	TB	TB (fit)
Haemoglobin(g/L)	130	120	125	145
RANGE	(110-150)	(90-140)	(110-180)	(120-180)
Haematocrit(L/L)	0.38	0.36	0.40	0.42
RANGE	(0.31-0.45)	(0.30-0.42)	(0.35-0.46)	(0.37-0.45)
RBC (x 10^{12}/L)	9.9	10.0	10.5	10.8
RANGE	(8.0-11.0)	(8.8-12.6)	(8.5-12.5)	(8.5-12.9)

MCV (fl)	41 -49	
MCHC (g/L)	310-370	(max value = saturated)
Platelets (x 10^9/L)	240-550	

WBC (x 10^9/L)	6.0-12.0	(often higher in yearlings)
Neutrophil (x 10^9/L)[%]*	2.7-6.7 [45-55%]	(higher in foals)
Lymphocyte (x 10^9/L)[%]	1.5-5.5 [35-50%]	(n:l :: 1.2:1.0)
Eosinophil (x 10^9/L)[%]	0.1-0.6 [0-5%]	
Monocyte (x 10 ^{9}/L)[%]	0.0-0.2 [0-3%]	

Bone Marrow M:E Ratio   0.5 : 1.0-1.5

(* Stab or unsegmented neutrophils are not usually present in normal blood)

[Note: i) normoblasts/reticulocytes do not often occur in peripheral blood.
ii) early erythrocytes may show Heinz Bodies]

$$MCV(fl) = \frac{Haematocrit}{RBC} \times 1000$$

$$MCHC(g/l) = \frac{Haemoglobin}{Haematocrit}$$

Note: These values are those which are regarded as normal in the Clinical Pathology Laboratory, Department of Veterinary Pathology, Leahurst.

B) Plasma and Serum Biochemistry:

Parameter (units)	Normal Value/Range
Total Protein (serum)(g/L)	62.5 - 70.0
Albumin (g/L)	27.0 - 36.5 (A/G x100 = 100%)
Globulin (g/L)	17.0 - 40.0 (8-32 in newborn)
α globulin	8.0 - 13.0
α₁globulin	2.0 - 4.0
α₂globulin	6.0 - 13.0
β globulin	8.0 - 15.0
β₁globulin	7.0 - 13.0
β₂globulin	6.0 - 10.0
γ globulin	7.0 - 14.0 (note foal IgG ex colostrum)
Fibrinogen (plasma)(g/L)	0.5 - 3.0

Bilirubin (Total) (μmol/L)	25 - 50 (up to 150 if starved >12 hrs)
Conj (Direct)(μmol/L)	4 - 15
Glucose (mmol/L)	3.5 - 6.0
Cholesterol (mmol/L)	2.5 - 3.5
Triglycerides(mmol/L)	0.1 - 0.4
Urea (mmol/L)	3.5 - 8.0
Creatinine (μmol/L)	90 - 200
Lactate (mmol/L)	0.6 - 1.9 (slightly lower in arterial blood)
Inorg Phos(mmol/L)	1.0 - 2.0 (higher in young: up to 4.0)
Bile Acids(μmol/l)	10 - 20

Calcium(Total)(mmol/L)	2.5 - 4.0
Calcium(ionised)(mmol/l)	1.5 - 1.8
Copper (μmol/L)	10 - 20
Sodium (mmol/L)	134 - 143
Potassium (mmol/L)	3.5 - 5.5
Potassium (red cell)(mmol/l)	85 - 115
Chloride (mmol/L)	90 - 105
Iron (μmol/l)	25 - 30
Iron binding cap (μmol/l)	40 - 80
Magnesium (mmol/l)	0.6 - 1.0

Ammonia (μmol/l)	< 40

Cortisol (nmol/L)	25 - 155 (marked diurnal variations)
T3 (nmol/L)	0.5 - 2.0
T4 (nmol/L)	4 - 40 (high in neonate)
Insulin (μIU/ml)	5 - 36
Parathormone (pmol/l)	60 - 80

Vitamin B₁₂ (pg/ml)	> 1000
Folate (ng/ml)	7 - 13

C) Acid - Base Balance:

	Arterial	Venous
pH	7.35 - 7.41	7.36 - 7.43
pCO_2	37 - 43	45 - 49
pO_2	73 - 98	36 - 47
HCO_3^- (mmol/L)	22.5 - 26.5	22.3 - 25.0
Base Excess	0 - +4	-2 - +1.5

Metabolic Fluid requirement = 15 ml / kg / day

$$Litres = \frac{bodyweight[Kg] \times dehydration[percent]}{100}$$

Bicarbonate Deficit (mls of 8.4%/molar) = 0.3 x Base excess x Body Weight (kg)

Note: Bicarbonate should only be administered when Base Excess is negative, pH is acidic and plasma bicarbonate is low - ie in metabolic acidosis. Bicarbonate is contraindicated in respiratory acidosis.

D) **Enzymes:**

Alkaline phosphatase (AlP)(iu/L)	< 250 (higher in young)
Aspartate aminotransferase(AST)(iu/L)	80 - 250
Creatine kinase (CK)(iu/L)	< 50
Lactate dehydrogenase(LDH)(iu/L)	76 - 400 (higher in young)
LDH$_1$ (% of total)	8 - 12
LDH$_2$ (% of total)	20 - 30
LDH$_3$ (% of total)	35 - 45
LDH$_4$ (% of total)	12 - 20
LDH$_5$ (% of total)	1 - 5
γ Glutamyl transpeptidase (γGT)(iu/L)	< 40
Glutamate dehydrogenase (GLDH)(iu/l)	< 6
Glutathione peroxidase(GsHPx)(m/mlRBC's)	> 40
Intestinal alk phos (IAlP) (iu/L)	< 30
Sorbitol dehydrogenase (SDH)(iu/L)	< 2*

* very short half-life in vitro and in vivo (< 2hrs)

Note: Alanine Aminotransferase estimation is of no practical/diagnostic value in the horse

E) Blood Coagulation:

Prothrombin Time (PT) (First Stage PT)	12 - 15 sec
Activated Prothrombin Time	9 - 12 sec
In vitro clotting time	5 - 7 mins
Bleeding Time (*in vivo*)	2 - 3 mins

F) Cerebrospinal Fluid:

COLLECT INTO PLAIN (Sterile) AND EDTA tubes

Colour	water clear
Cisternal pressure	150-300 mm H_2O
Refractive Index	1.334-1.335
Ph	7.4
Cell Count (Total)	< 0.005 x 10^9/L
Cell Distribution	Neutrophils and small lymphocytes only
Protein (total)	< 1.0 g/L
Pandey Test (Globulins)*	NEGATIVE
Creatine Kinase#	< 2 iu/L
Glucose	50-60% of blood glucose
Asp. Transaminase (AST)	< 20 iu/L
Lactic dehydrogenase(LDH)	< 8 iu/l

* **Note: Pandey Test using concentrated Phenol**
# **CK may be higher [30 - 50 iu/l] in foals < 7 days old.**
Note: Cells in CSF degenerate fast... assay < 15 min!

G) Synovial Fluid:

COLLECT INTO PLAIN (Sterile) AND EDTA tubes.

If bacterial culture required collect into BLOOD CULTURE TUBES

Appearance	Clear, non turbid, pale yellow
Volume	Variable with joint
Viscosity (Stringing test)	POSITIVE
Leucocyte Count (Total)	$< 0.5 \times 10^9/L$
Total Protein	$< 18 \text{ g/L}$

Note: normal synovial fluid clots with acetic acid!

H) Peritoneal / Pleural Fluid:

COLLECT INTO PLAIN (Sterile) AND EDTA tubes

Colour	Clear, Pale yellow, non clotting
Protein	$< 20 \text{ g/L}$
Leucocyte Count (Total)	$< 1 \times 10^9/L$
Total red cell count	negligible

Note:
i) Peritoneal fluid which has the same PCV as jugular blood is probably from a blood vessel.
ii) Peritoneal fluid with a very high PCV is likely to have come from the spleen.
iii) Peritoneal fluid with a PCV slightly less than jugular blood may indicate peritoneal bleeding.
iv) Peritoneal fluid with a very low PCV is probably the result of a strangulating lesion.

I) Urine:

Collect into sterile containers (ensure bottles etc are clean and free from sugar contamination)

pH	7.5 - 9.5
Colour	clear or cloudy/turbid
Deposit	Carbonate crystals
Blood	NEGATIVE
SG	1.020 - 1.060

NOTE: *Normal equine urine may be markedly cloudy due to high calcium carbonate content. Initial flow of urine may be clear with a heavy deposit passed at the end of the flow. Normal equine urine is also usually markedly viscid.*

10

NOTES:

REPRODUCTIVE DATA
Seasonal Breeder -- Spring and Summer

1) MARE:

Oestrus cycle length   13 - 25 days (normal = 21 days)

In oestrus for   2 - 7 days (normal = 4 days)

Ovulation occurs 24 - 48 hrs **before** end of behavioural oestrus

Gestation length   320 - 360 days (normal 335 - 340 days)

Plasma hormone concentrations:

	OESTRONE Conjugated (total) (ng/ml)	PROGESTERONE (nmol/l)	eCG (PMSG)
Early Oestrus	< 6.0	< 3.0	-ve
Late Oestrus	< 6.0	< 3.0	
Luteal Phase	< 6.0	> 12	-ve
Pregnancy :			
8 - 25 days	< 6.0	> 13 - 57	-ve
40 - 100 days	< 6.0	> 10.0	+ve(#)
100 - 150 days	< 6.0	< 1.0	-ve
200 - 300 days	6 - 200+	< 1.0	-ve
300 - term	> 6.0	< 1.0	-ve
Prolonged Dioestrus		13 - 57	

	OESTROGEN (pg/ml)	PROGESTERONE (ng/ml)	TESTOSTERONE (nmol/L)
Granulosa Cell Tumour	-	-	> 0.5

\# = false negatives may occur before 60 days and after 90 days)

Urinary Hormone Concentrations:

	Total Urinary Oestrogens (nmol/l)
LUTEAL PHASE	< 500
FOLLICULAR PHASE	600 - 3000
PREGNANCY (over 100 days)	> 3000

NOTES

2) STALLION

Semen characteristics:

Volume	50 - 200 ml
Gel-free volume	35 - 100 ml
pH	7.3 - 7.7

Product of:

sperm conc x gel-free volume x % progressive motile sperm x % morphologically normal sperm for a stallion with a book of 40 mares should exceed:

1100×10^6 (September - January)

1700×10^6 (February - April)

2000×10^6 (May)

2200×10^6 (June)

1700×10^6 (July and August)

Plasma hormone concentrations:
(see also TEST FOR CRYPTORCHIDISM: p19)

	Conjugated Oestrone (ng/ml)	Testosterone (nmol/l)
Stallion	10 - 50	5.0 - 30.0
False Rig	< 0.02	0.03 - 0.15 0.05 - 0.19 (after hCG)
True Rig	0.1 - 10	0.3 - 4.3 1.0 - 12.9 (after hCG)

Hormone values by courtesy of SERONO LABORATORIES

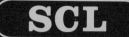

DIAGNOSTIC TESTS

i) Bromosulphthalein Clearance Test:

Procedure: Starve horse for 12 hours
Collect two initial samples at 30 minute intervals.
Inject 1 g BSP IV (2.2 mg/kg).
Collect blood samples at 1 minute intervals for 5-10 minutes.

NORMAL VALUE FOR BSP CLEARANCE $(T^1/_2)$ = 125 - 200 secs.

Note: BSP Retention can be determined following administration of an accurately calculated dose of BSP (5 mg/kg) from one sample taken at 15 minutes. Normal animals should have a negligible percentage of the initial concentration remaining at this time.

ii) Glucose Absorbtion Test:

Procedure: Collect Blood Samples into Fl ox tubes 30 minutes and 60 minutes prior to start of test (STAT samples) (best if unstressed) (In-dwelling IV cannula).
Administer 1 g glucose/Kg Body Weight as 10% solution by stomach tube. Take blood sample (Fl oxalate anticoagulant) immediately after glucose administration and at 30 minute intervals for 3 hours.

Note: Xylose absorbtion test is identical but uses 5 g Xylose per kg body weight given as 5% solution by stomach tube.

NORMAL VALUE FOR GLUCOSE/XYLOSE ABSORBTION = peak at 90-120 mins at 2x basal conc.

iii) <u>Sodium Sulphanilate Clearance Test</u>:

<u>Procedure</u>:

Collect blood samples (plain) 5 minutes before and immediately before administration of 10 mg/kg Na sulphanilate by slow IV. Sample immediately (stat) and at 30 minute intervals for 2 hours.

Calculate $T^1/_2$.

NORMAL VALUE FOR SODIUM SULPHANILATE CLEARANCE = 35-45 min

iv) <u>Zinc Sulphate Turbidity Test</u>:

<u>Procedure</u>:

Prepare a solution of Zinc Sulphate (205mg in 1 litre boiled distilled water).

Introduce 6 ml of the solution into 7 or 10 ml Vacutainer (Becton-Dickinson Ltd, UK) in such a way that some vacuum still remains. [The solution would otherwise disssolve atmospheric CO_2 to form a milky suspension of zinc carbonate]. These containers may be kept almost indefinitely.

Add 0.1 ml foal serum to the tube and mix gently. Leave for 60 minutes. Read by holding tube up to the print below. If you can read the print size the globulin level is as shown opposite to the print.

Note: A rough qualitative assessment may be made at 10 minutes when <u>obvious turbidity</u> = <u>adequate globulin</u>).

Zinc sulphate turbidity test   = < 3 g /l

Zinc Sulphate Turbidity Test   =   3 - 6 g /l

Zinc Sulphate Turbidity Test   = 6 - 8 g /l

Zinc Sulphate Turbidity Test   = > 8 g/l

v) **Cryptorchidism**:

Procedure:

In horses < 2 years old and donkeys of any age. Clotted blood sample obtained immediately prior to administration of 6,000 iu human chorionic gonadotrophin (IV).
Second sample obtained 30 - 120 min later.

Samples submitted for testosterone analysis.
In horses 3 years old or older a single sample of clotted blood submitted for oestrone sulphate analysis is sufficient.

Expected values:

	Testosterone (nmol/l)		Oestrone Sulphate (ng/l)
	Before	After	
Entire male	-	-	10 - 50
Cryptorchid	0.3 - 4.3	**1.0 - 12.9**	0.1 - 10
Gelding	0.3 - 0.15	**0.05 - 0.19**	< 0.02

vi) **Paracentesis abdominis**:

Procedure:
Clip/prepare midline, midway between umbilicus and xiphoid (most dependent part).
Either
  a) use 19 g 2" hypodermic needle thrust through linea alba. Twist and withdraw slightly and/or turn hub to encourage flow

OR
  b) Use guarded No 11 scalpel blade to make stab incision through skin to depth of about 1cm into linea alba. Carefully thrust teat cannula through linea.

Collect into EDTA and plain and sterile plain tubes (twisting needle/cannula often helps).
Assess colour, viscosity, clarity immediately. Submit to lab for cytology and protein analysis (if required sterile sample for bacteriology).

vii) **Paracentesis thoracis**:

Procedure:
Prepare site on **both** sides (always tap both) at 7-9th I-C space at level of point of shoulder.
Local analgesia and stab incision in skin. Use trochar and canula or 10 g iv catheter, or 16 g needle as appropriate (all with three way tap or one way (Heimlich) valve. Insert off anterior edge of rib.

Collect into sterile plain, EDTA and plain tubes.
Assess quantity, colour, clarity, odour immediately. Submit to lab for cytology, bacteriology and protein analysis.

viii) **Transtracheal wash**:

Procedure:

Clip/prepare site ($^2/_3$ down mid ventral neck). Local analgesia (5 - 10 ml). Pass wide gauge (>12) cannula between rings into trachea (downward). Pass long flexible catheter (eg dog urinary catheter) downwards until cough induced. Introduce 20 - 40 ml sterile PBS. Immediately aspirate while withdrawing catheter slightly.

Collect sample in plain sterile, EDTA and plain tubes.
Submit to lab for bacteriology, cytology.

Note: do not use a needle as a cannula... it may cut the catheter in half!

ix) **Bronchio-alveolar lavage**:

Procedure:

Standing sedation (Butorphenol useful). Pass BAL catheter (BAL Catheter, Bivona, USA) (available from Irish Equine Centre, Johnstown, Naas, Co Kildare, Ireland) into trachea (via nasal meatus). Introduce as far as possible to wedge in airway (inflate cuff if present). Introduce 100-300 00ml sterile phosphate buffered saline (PBS) under pressure. Withdraw fluid into sterile plain, plain and edta tubes.

Submit for cytology, bacteriology

NORMAL washings contain alveolar macrophages, few degenerate neutrophils, epithelial/alveolar cells

NOTE: Cease if coughing severe. May be performed using sheathed BAL catheter using an endoscope or via endoscope introduced until wedged.

(x) **Bone Marrow Biopsy**:

Procedure:
Full asepsis essential. Best site = mid line mid sternum (cortex thin).
Alternative sites : Wing of ilium, rib (both difficult). Use marrow punch and aspirate using 20 ml syringe. AVOID excessive pressure for long periods. Large blood flow undesirable.
Collect into EDTA (with egg albumin) and make smear immediately (fix imediately with alcohol). Stain Geimsa (1:100 24 hours OR Leishmans).

(xi) **Liver Biopsy**:

Procedure:
Full asepsis essential. RIGHT SIDE. Best site = centre of quadrangle formed by:
  a) line from point of elbow to point of hip
  b) line from point of shoulder to point of hip
  c) 13th rib
  d) 10th rib

Local analgesia of skin and intercostal muscles and pleura. Stab incision with No 11 blade adjacent to cranial edge of rib (BLOOD VESSELS ALONG CAUDAL EDGE). Insert Tru-Cut biopsy instrument horizontally and through pleural space on expiration. feel each anatomical layer. Liver capsule is firm and liver usually denser than other tissues.
NOTE: Bleeding disorders checked first. If chosen site further back then instrument needs to be angled progressively moredown ward and forward and length of instrument needs to be longer.
Biopsy taken at the 14th intercostal space requires that instrument is aimed at opposite elbow.

xii) **Renal Clearance Ratios**:

Procedure:
Obtain simultaneous venous blood and urine (preferably by catheterisation).

a) **Creatinine clearance ratio ($\propto$ to GFR):**
Values derived from the formula (expressed in %)

$$\text{Creatinine Clearance (GFR)} = \frac{[\text{Creatinine}]_{serum}}{[\text{Creatinine}]_{urine}}$$

(NORMAL = 1.0 - 2.0 ml/kg/min)

Note: difficult test due to problem in obtaining total 24 hour urine.

b) **Electrolyte clearance ratio:**

$$\text{Clearance for [X]} = \frac{[\text{Creatinine}]_{serum}}{[\text{Creatinine}]_{urine}} \quad X \quad \frac{[X]_{urine}}{[X]_{serum}} \quad X \ 100\%$$

Clearance Ratios:

Na^+	=	0.1 - 1.0%
K^+	=	35 - 55%
Ca^{2+}	=	1.5 - 3.5%
PO_4^{3-}	=	0.0 - 0.5%
Cl^-	=	0.05 - 1.5%

Note: Simultaneously obtained urine and plasma samples - accuracy dependent on normal renal function. If renal function not normal test is invalid (renal creatinine clearance ratio not normal). Values may show diurnal variation - results used as a guide rather than absolute.

c) **Excretion Factors:**

$$\frac{[\text{Urine concentration(mmol/l)}] \ X \ 0.04}{\text{Urine Specific Gravity} - 0.997}$$

Calcium excretion = 15 μmol/mosmol (micromoles per milliosmole)

Phosphate excretion = 15 μmol/mosmol

(xiii) **ACTH Response and Dexamethasone Supression Test**:

Procedure:

2 DAY METHOD	1 DAY METHOD
Time 0:Collect blood (CORTISOL)	Time 0:Collect blood (CORTISOL)
Inject 40μg/kg Dexamethasone (IM)	Inject 10mg Dexamethasone (IM)
4 hrs: Blood (CORTISOL)	3 hrs: Blood (CORTISOL)
24 hrs:Blood (CORTISOL)	Inject 1 mg ACTH IV
Inject ACTH gel (1U/kg, IM)	5 hrs: Blood (CORTISOL)
36 hrs:Collect (CORTISOL)	

Interpretation: **2 day test**: NORMAL: Cortisol falls to 30% of baseline in 4 hours and remains at 30% for 24 hours. Then 2-3x elevation by 8-12 hrs after injection of ACTH.

1 day test: Cortisol depressed to 35% baseline by 3 hours then rise to 2.5x base at 5 hours

NOTE: Pituitary adenoma also confirmed by IV 1 mg thyrotropin-releasing hormone (TSH)--> rise in CORTISOL at 30 minutes. Also by INSULIN estimation (> 100ug/ml) and no response to IV glucose challenge.

xiv) **Thyroid Stimulation Test**

Procedure:
Blood sample (plain) obtained 2 and 0 hours before start. Inject (IV) 5iu THYROTROPIN (SIGMA Chemicals LTD). Plain blood samples at 1, 2, 4, 6, 8 hours post injection. Submitted for T_3 and T_4 estimation (SERONO LABORATORIES)

NORMAL: Peak increase of T_3 at 4 hours post injection. Little change in T_4.

NOTE: Most available TSH is of BOVINE ORIGIN. THIS SHOULD NOT BE USED IN VIVO IN HORSES due to risk of transmitted CNS disorders and MUST NOT BE USED for horses intended for human consumption. (Clarification of the risks are expected in due course). Where practicable HUMAN origin TSH or thyrotropin releasing hormone may be used. THESE ARE VERY EXPENSIVE.

NOTES:

NOTES

ELECTROCARDIOGRAPHIC DATA:

Most useful lead configuration is BASE - APEX (less affected by movement and respiration):

Right Arm - Right jugular groove ⅓rd up neck
Left Arm - Left thorax at apex beat (Intercostal space 6)
Right Leg - EARTH (any place remote eg withers)

    i) Record 1 mv standard (ensure sensitivity is lowest possible)

    ii) Select speed (25mm/sec) - useful to have one section at 50mm/sec

    ii) SELECT LEAD I - RUN

Normal values:

		P wave Duration (msec)	P-R Interval (msec)	QRS Duration (msec)	Q-T Interval (msec)
Horses	Mean	140	330	130	510
	Range	(80-200)	220-560	80-170	320-640
Ponies	Mean	100	217	78	462
	Range	85-106	209-226	66-86	420-483

(Reference: Hilwig R.W., 1987)

NOTE: Superimposed 50mHz pattern from mains lights (Flourescent tubes etc).
EARTH electrode important
Ensure good gel/spirit contact

INTERPRETATION:
    1) PULSE RATE =   /min, HEART RATE =   /min : PULSE DEFICIT: YES/NO
    2) JUGULAR PULSE : YES/NO;   MUCOUS MEMBRANE COLOUR:
    3) CRT =   sec
    4) GENERALISED SIGNS OF CHF? YES/NO
        a) Is there a P for every QRS?
        b) Is there a QRS for every P?
        c) Are all the complexes the same?
        d) Are F waves present?
        e) Any pauses/irregularities
        f) Any S-T slurring/depression

KEEP ACCURATE RECORDS AND RELEVANT ECG TRACE
    - CLEARLY IDENTIFIED/DATED with technical data written onto trace

28

NOTES

NOTES

30

NOTES

NOTES

INDEX OF DRUGS USED IN EQUINE MEDICINE

PRESCRIPTIONS

NOTE: Good prescription principles include:

i) Write legibly and sign with your normal signature
ii) Use approved names for drugs IN CAPITAL LETTERS - DO NOT ABBREVIATE
iii) State duration of treatment (where known)
iv) Write out microgram / nanogram (DO NOT ABBREVIATE)
v) Always put a 0 before a decimal point.
vi) GIVE PRECISE INSTRUCTIONS concerning ROUTE/DOSE
vii) Any alterations invalidate the prescription - rewrite.
viii) Prescriptions for CONTROLLED DRUGS must be entirely handwritten.

Abbreviations commonly used in prescriptions:

ac	-before meals	prn	-as needed
ad (s)	-right ear (left)	qd	-every day
au	-both ears	qid	-four times daily
ad lib	-at pleasure	qod	-every other day
amp	-ampoule	q 4h	-every 4 hours (etc)
aq	-water	qA	-sufficient quantity
bid	-twice daily	rep	-repeat
c	-with	s	-without
cap(s)	-capsules	sid	-once daily
circ	-about,approx	sig	-instruction/label
disp	-dispense	solve	-dissolve
et	-and	sol'n	-solution
ext	-extract	SC	-subcutaneously
g	-gram	SS	-half
gtt(s)	-drop(s)	stat	-immediately
IM(im)	-intramuscularly	susp	-suspension
IV(iv)	-intravenously	tabs	-tablets
id	-the same	tbs	-tablespoon
m	-mix	tid	-three times daily
mcg(μg)	-microgram	tr	-tincture
mg	-milligram	tsp	-teaspoon
ml	-milliliter	Ut dict	-as directed
non rep.	-do not repeat	(s)	-left
o.d. (s)	-right eye (left)	(d)	-right
o.m.	-every morning		
o.n.	-every evening		
o.u.	-both eyes		
pc	-after meals		
po	-by mouth		

Note: Avoid using the specific administration abbreviations qd, qod, sid, bid, tid because they may be confused with other abbreviations and are almost unknown outside the vet profession. If you are in any doubt write out plain directions in longhand!

DRUG CATEGORIZATION FOR PRESCRIPTION PURPOSES

GSL: A preparation which falls in the General Sales List ie may be sold by anyone over the counter in any appropriate retail shop.

P: A pharmacy prepared medicine which can be sold by a retail pharmacy or veterinarian.

PML: Schedule 1, Medicines Order 1985. Specially listed veterinary products which may be sold by pharmacists or agricultural merchants or supplied by veterinarians.

POM: May only be dispensed/sold with a prescription. Veterinary Surgeons who dispense drugs from their own stocks for *treatment of animals under their care* are deemed to have prescribed the drugs (provided that the correct labelling and packaging has been used).

CD: Controlled Drugs are regulated by the Misuse of Drugs Act 1971 and the Misuse of Drugs Regulations, 1985. These associated regulations classify the controlled drugs into 5 schedules numbered in decreasing order of severity of control.

Schedule 1: LSD, Heroine, and other opiates **Not applicable to veterinary use**

Schedule 2: Includes Morphine, Pethidine, Papaveretum, LA/SA Immobilon, Methadone etc.
Record all purchases and keep in a bound record. Also record each individual dispense within 24 hours. Records must be kept for 2 calender years after the last entry is made.

Drugs must be kept in a locked container. **You could be prosecuted for failure to comply with this act.**

Schedule 3: Includes buprenorphine, pentazocine, phenobarbitone, pentobarbitone.
Receipts of requisition only to be kept.

Schedule 4: Includes butorphanol, benzodiazepines.
Exempted from control when used in normal veterinary practice eg

Schedule 5: Preparations containing codeine, cough medicines etc.
Exempted from control,

Note: Prescriptions for Schedule 2 and 3 Controlled Drugs MUST be written in longhand by the prescribing veterinarian. It is NOT acceptable to use typewriting or the handwriting of any other person.
NOTE: Most drugs have established withdrawal times. These MUST be considered when using drugs to treat horses intended for human consumption.

NOTES:

SECTION 1: *Drugs acting on* CENTRAL NERVOUS SYSTEM:

a) CNS/Respiratory stimulants:

Doxapram Hydrochloride: POM
  Dopram-V [*Willows Francis Veterinary*]

  Indications: Respiratory stimulation (drug induced respiratory depression / neonatal)
  (**not** muscle relaxant-induced depression).

  Forms: 20 ml multi-dose vials (20 mg/ml) for injection.

  Dose: 0.5 - 1.0 mg/kg IV depending on response. Dose adjusted for depth of anaesthesia / degree
  of respiratory depression.

  Notes: Seldom indicated in adults. Short duration. Respiratory rate/tidal volume slightly
  increased. Antagonises opiate induced respiratory depression (without affecting analgesia). Repeat
  doses not administered until first worn off and repeat dose indicated. May cause arousal in
  anesthetised horses.
  Excessive doses may produce hyperventilation (reduced pCO_2, cerebral vasoconstriction,
  hypoxia - possible brain damage).
  High doses during (or following) anaesthesia with halogenated hydrocarbons may produce cardiac
  arrhythmias.

b) Analgesics

Butorphenol Tartrate: POM/CD (S-IV)
   Torbugesic [*C-VET LTD*]

Indications: Relief of musculoskeletal and visceral pain (colic). With sedative / tranquilliser for standing sedation / restraint.

Forms: 50 ml multidose bottle - 10 mg/ml for injection.

Dose: 0.1 mg/kg IV

Notes: Unlikely to cause excitement after intravenous injection.

Etorphine Hydrochloride: POM/CD (S-11)
   Large Animal Immobilon (with acepromazine) [*C-VET LTD*]

Indications: Reversible neuroleptanalgesia (narcosis with analgesia), restraint minor surgical interventions.

Forms: Yellow aqueous solution 2.45mg/ml (2.25 mg/ml etorphine base) with acepromazine maleate BP (Vet) 10mg/ml
(Marketed with **diprenorphine** (qv) (*Revivon*).

Dose: 0.5ml/50kg (minimum) IV or IM. Effect approx 45 min (if longer period **essential** additional half dose IV). IM injection causes marked excitement + long, inco-ordinated inductions.

Notes: Equal volume Revivon (total volume Immobilon) IV as soon as possible after procedure completed. Recover with minimum disturbance and noise. Muscular tremors common (may diminish if left recumbent for a few minutes). Possible tranquillisation after reversal.
High risk in old / debilitated animals - precautionary procedures, eg maintenance of airway is vital.
Tachy- or brady- cardia, hyper- or hypo- tension, and severe respiratory depression always occur.
Risk of respiratory depression in neonate when given to parturient mare.
NOT for horses with cardiac arrhythmias, history of endocarditis, or liver damage.
Entero-hepatic re-cycling may cause excitement and "walking" six to eight hours after recovery (close supervision essential) (reversed with a further half dose of Revivon (possibly prevented by extra half dose of Revivon sc).
Paraphimosis may be seen as a sequel to priapism in horses.
Safety of personnel paramount.
Prepare NALOXONE before handling (LEGAL /MORAL REQUIREMENT; p54)
Dispose needles/syringes with extreme care!

Flunixin meglumine: (See p97)

Methindizate: POM
Isaverin (with dipyrone) [*Bayer UK*]

Indications: Spasmolytic and intestinal analgesic used in relief of spasmodic colic pain.

Forms: Yellowish aqueous solution for injection (250 mg /ml), 100 ml multidose vials.

Dose: 10 mg/kg IV q8h pnr

Notes: NOT for SC or IM use. Maximum effect after 10 - 20 min

Methadone: POM/CD (SII)
Physeptone [*Calmic Medical*]

Indications: Relief of musculoskeletal pain. Useful with sedative tranquillizers for standing
sedation.

Forms: Single dose 1 ml ampoules (10 mg/ml / 50 mg/ml).

Dose: 30 - 40 mg IV / 500 kg

Notes: Can cause some excitement eg. box walking, but less marked than   with morphine.

Morphine Sulphate: POM/CD (S-II)
Morphine Sulphate [*Evans*]

Indications: Relief of severe musculoskeletal pain (esp long bone fractures). Used in sedative
"cocktails".

Forms: Single dose vial - 10mg/ml or 60mg/ml.

Dose: 0.02 - 0.1 mg/kg IM/IV, 20 ml multidose vial for injection

Notes: Excitement/box-walking in normal pain-free horses.
Must be kept in a separate, locked receptacle, and purchase and dispensing registered.

Pethidine:

Pethidine BP [*Arnolds*]

<u>Indications</u>: Relief of musculoskeletal and gastro-enteric pain. Effective spasmolytic. Useful in combination with acepromazine and/or xylazine for standing sedation.

<u>Forms</u>: Multi-dose vials - 50 mg/ml for injection.

<u>Dose</u>: 2mg/kg (1g / 500 kg IM or slow IV).

<u>Notes</u>: May cause excitement / profuse sweating if IV - better IM (rapid distribution)

<u>Xylazine</u>: (See p43)

c) Tranquilisers and sedatives

Acepromazine Maleate:
  ACP [*Boots*], Berkace [*Berk*])

Indications: Restraint, control of excitement, premedication. Examination of penis.

Forms: 10 mg/ml, 10 ml, 20ml and 50 ml solution for injection. Multidose bottles.
    25 mg tablet for oral use.

Dose: Injection : 0.04 - 0.11 mg / kg IV/IM/SC (for premed use lower doses)
    Oral : 0.1 - 0.2 mg/kg (slow / variable effect)

Notes: **Contraindicated in hypotensive conditions**; Acute hypotension resulting from ACP may
be treated with phenylephrine or norepinephrine.
May cause penile prolapse/priapism/paraphimosis (especially entire stallions).
Significant drug interactions with Quinidine Sulphate (cardiac depression and hypotension).
NB: 2mg/kg sol. also available (CHECK STRENGTH).

Chloral hydrate BVetC
  Chloral Hydrate [*E R Squibb*]

Indications: Sedative-hypnotic. Little effect on reflexes, blood pressure and respiration.

Forms: Crystalline powder

Dose: 65-110 mg/kg IV (10%) or PO (10%) via stomach tube.
    (Usual dose for a 450kg horse is 50-60g).

Notes: Cheap. Severe reactions / sloughing if extravascular.
Irritant to mucous membranes at > 5%, Unpleasant taste (restrict all other water for up to 24
hours before drink voluntarily). Delayed affect after administration due to required metabolism.
Additive effect if used with other CNS drugs.

Detomidine   POM
    Demosodan [*Norden*]

Indications: Sedation and analgesia, premedication

Forms: Solution for IV/IM injection 10 mg/ml (5 ml and 20 ml multidose vial)

Dose: Level of sedation

	Light	Medium	Heavy
Dosage(μg/kg)	10-20	20-40	40-80
Onset of effect	3-5 min	2-5 min	1-5 min
Duration	0.5-1 hr	0.5-1 hr	0.5-2 hr

Use 20 μg/kg for anaesthetic regime with ketamine @ 2.2 mg/kg 2-5 minutes later (P36)

Notes: Hypotensive if used alone. Marked bradycardia.
IM dose 1.5 - 2 X IV dose. Intractable horses sedated with sub-lingual dose use high dose and be prepared to wait.
Beware when using with sympathomimetic amines. Do NOT use in last trimester of pregnancy.
DO NOT USE WITH potentiated sulphonamides (fatal dysrrhythmias).
Maximal effects obtained when horse is left quiet after administration.
May be combined with butorphanol for good standing sedation.
Standing Sedation: **Detomidine** 10 μg/kg + **Butorphanol** 0.025mg/kg iv
    eg 0.5ml detomidine with 1.25ml butorphanol

Xylazine: POM
    Rompun [*Bayer*], Anased [*BK Pharmaceuticals*]

Indications: Sedative / intestinal analgesic with muscle relaxant effects. Premedication.

Presentation: 20 mg/ml (20ml multidose vial) for injection
               100 mg/ml (10 ml multidose vial) for injection
               500 mg dry powder (10 ml single dose vial)-diluent supplied

Dose: 0.5 - 1.1 mg/kg IV (slow)

Notes: Marked local reaction and unreliable effect IM (2- 3x IV dose).
1°/2° heart blocks common. Bradycardia pronounced / reduced cardiac output may cause hypotension. Hyperglycaemia and sweating.
Sedation lasts longer than analgesia. Somatic analgesia POOR, use local and/or systemic analgesic eg butorphanol for painful procedures.
Ensure correct solution used to calculate dose.

d) Anaesthetic agents:

<u>I) VOLATILE and GASEOUS AGENTS</u>:

<u>Halothane</u>:   POM
    Fluothane [*Pitman-Moore*], Halothane [*Hoechst*]

    <u>Indications</u>: Maintenance of anaesthesia. Induction in foals.

    <u>Forms</u>: Colourless volatile liquid with characteristic sweet smell.

    <u>Dose</u>: Normally 1.5 - 3% used for maintenance (dependent on other agents and circuits used)

    <u>Notes</u>: Potent cardiovascular depressant (GREAT CARE).

<u>Isofluorane</u>:   POM
    Aerane [*Abbott*]

    <u>Indications</u>: Maintenance of anaesthesia. Induction in foals.

    <u>Forms</u>: Colourless volatile liquid with pungent unpleasant smell.

    <u>Dose</u>: As for halothane

    <u>Notes</u>: Least effect on cardiovascular system of volatile agents. Low solubility gives rapid induction and recovery (ideal agent for foals). Expensive. USE WITH CARE!

<u>Nitrous Oxide</u>:   POM

    <u>Indications</u>: Maintenance of general anaesthesia. Weak analgesic. Useful support for volatile agents.

    <u>Forms</u>: Colourless, sweet-smelling gas in cylinders (BLUE).

    <u>Dose</u>: **Never** exceed 50% mixture with oxygen. Use high flow, semi-closed circle systems.

    <u>Notes</u>: Care in heavy horses in dorsal recumbency (only safe if oxygenation can be monitored using arterial blood gas analysis or oximetry). Second gas effect useful at induction. Diffusion hypoxia - possible harmful effect.

II) INTRAVENOUS AGENTS:

Alphoxalone/alphadolone: POM
  Saffan [*Pitman Moore*], Althesin [*Pitman Moore*)

  <u>Indications</u>: Short acting anaesthetic for foals

  <u>Forms</u>: Oily solution (12mg total steroid /ml) for injection, 20 ml multi/single dose vials (cannot be stored open or resealed)

  <u>Dose</u>: 2 - 5 mg (total steroid) /kg rapid IV

  <u>Notes</u>: Safe, short acting (< 10 min). Very expensive. Can be repeated as required or infused continuously.

Etorphine:see Analgesics (p)

Ketamine: POM
  Vetalar [*Parke Davis*], Ketaset [*C Vet*]

  <u>Indications</u>: Short duration general anaesthesia **with xylazine or detomidine. (GGE or valium may also be used)**.

  <u>Forms</u>: 10 ml multi-dose vials, 100 mg/ml

  <u>Dose</u>: 2 - 2.2 mg/kg IV.

  <u>Notes</u>: **Never administer ketamine alone or first!** (Ensure pre-filled syringes are clearly labelled).

Methohexitone: POM/CD (S-II)
  Brietal [*Eli Lilly*]

  Indications: Anesthetic induction.

  Forms: 2.5 g powder in 250 ml vial/ 250 ml diluent supplied- use 1% or 2.5% solution.

  Dose: 5 - 10 mg /kg IV bolus.
       (1g / 180 kg with light premedication.
       1 g / 360 kg with heavy premedication).

  Notes: Rapid, ultra short-acting. Irritant perivenously - catheter preferred.
  Do not reconstitute with Hartmans/Ringer Lactate. Use solutions within 24 hours.

Propofol: POM
  Rapinovet [*Coopers*]

  Indications: Induction of anaesthesia in foals/small ponies.

  Forms: White emulsion (10mg/ml), single use 20 ml vials

  Dose: 2 mg/kg IV

  Notes: Rapidly metabolised, short acting. Expensive.

Thiopentone Sodium: POM/CD (S-II)
  Intraval Sodium [*Rhone Merieux*], Thiopentone Sodium [*IMS, UK Ltd*]

  Indications: Anaesthetic induction, short duration procedures.

  Forms: Dry powder reconstituted to 2.5%, 5% or 10% solution - diluent provided.

  Dose: 10 - 15 mg/kg (1g/90kg) with **light** premedication.
       7 - 10 mg/kg (1g/180kg) with **heavy** premedication.

  Notes: **Do not reconstitute with Hartmans or Ringer Lactate.**
  Extremely alkaline- very irritant perivascularly, use of catheter preferred. Immediate action if
  perivascular injection suspected (using copious amounts of saline +/- lignocaine HCl). Always
  dilute solution to 50-60 ml.

e) Anticonvulsants:

Diazepam: POM/CD (SIV)
   Valium [*Roche*]

   Indications: Anticonvulsant, sedative, muscle relaxant. Useful sedative /muscle relaxant and premedicant in foals.

   Presentation: Solution for injection 5mg/ml in 10ml single dose vials.

   Dose: Pre-anaesthetic: 0.05 - 0.4 mg/kg IV (average 0.22mg/kg).
      Status epilepticus: up to 1mg/kg (slow IV)

   Notes: Unacceptable ataxia if given alone to adult horses.
   Use slow IV injection (>1 min / 10mg).
   Causes thrombophlebitis. Minimal cardiovascular effects.
   Do not dilute or mix with other agents (may be mixed with ketamine provided used immediately).
   If using infusion tubing inject as close to vein as possible. Avoid i/m.
   May replace GGE in induction regimes (esp foals).

Midazolam: POM/CD (S-IV)
   Hypnovel [*Roche*]

   Indications: As for diazepam (anticonvulsant activities)

   Forms: 10mg in 2mls vials

   Doses: As for diazepam. Dose titrated against the response.

   Notes: Short-acting benzodiazepine. Not yet evaluated in foals.
      Can be mixed with other agents.   Does not cause thrombophlebitis.

Pentobarbitone: POM/CD (S-II)
   Sagatal [*May Baker*]

   Indications: Sedation or anaesthesia of convulsive foals.

   Forms: Aqueous solution for injection (60 mg /ml) in 100 ml multidose vials.

   Dose: 15 - 20 mg /kg iv OR 2-10 mg/kg iv for acute anticonvulsive therapy, pnr

   Notes: Irritant (catheter obligatory). Not for anaesthesia of adult horses (much slower induction - more excitement).
   Do not use euthanasia solutions (200 mg/ml) for anaesthesia.

Phenytoin: POM
Epanutin [*Parke Davis*]

Indications: Anticonvulsive therapy in foals

Forms: Aqueous solution for IV injection 50 mg/ml
25mg and 100mg capsules for oral dosing

Dose: 5 - 10 mg/kg initial dose followed by 1 - 5 mg/kg q 2-4h (reducing after 12 hours to q 6-12 h IV / PO pnr

Notes: Reduce dosage according to effect. Prolonged high doses may cause hepatic failure.

Primidone: POM
Mysoline [*ICI*]

Indications: Anticonvulsive therapy in foals

Forms: 250 mg tablet for oral dosing

Dose: 2 g PO for 50 kg foal as loading dose, then 1 g q 12h

Notes: Long term use may result in tolerance and/or hepatopathy

f) Muscle relaxants:

Dantrolene Sodium: POM
Dantrium [*Norwich Eaton*]

Indications: Direct acting skeletal muscle relaxant. Prevention or treatment of myopathy (post-anaesthesia or exertional rhabdomyolysis)

Presentation: 100 mg caps for ORAL use

Dose: 10 mg /kg PO loading dose, 3 - 5 mg/kg PO q 1h
As prophylactic - full loading dose 60 minutes before surgery
Use cautiously before surgery (not fully evaluated)

Glyceryl Guaicolate BP: POM
GGE, Guaicol Glycerol Ether [*Sigma Chemical Company*], Guaifenesin, Gujatal*

Indications: Spinally acting muscle relaxant

Forms: White crystaline powder (* "Ready made" 10% solution available soon)
Home made - dissolve 50g powder in 500mls 5% dextrose or saline solution. Very difficult to dissolve. Helps to warm solution.

Dose: 20 - 50 mg /kg IV slowly until desired effect is attained.
     (ie approx half body wight in mls of 10% sloution, as a guide)

Notes: May precipitate out of solution, if very cold. Best to make up fresh. Also used as an expectorant (PO) (doubtful efficacy).

Very irritant perivascularly - if suspected infiltrate with large volumes of saline solution.
DO NOT USE FOR CASTING ONLY... no analgesic/anaesthetic properties!

Suxamethonium: POM
Scoline [*Roche*]

Indications: Depolarising muscle relaxant. Can be useful adjunct to injectable euthanasia.
Classically used as part of anaesthetic induction technique.

Forms: White water soluble powder reconstituted for injection.

Dose: 0.1 - 0.2 mg/kg IV.

Notes: Muscle fasciculations seen early. Short action. Muscle fasciculations present early.
Inactive in alkaline solution --DO NOT mix with barbiturates in syringe!

g) Parasympathomimetics

Neostigmine:
  Neostigmine [*Roche*]

  <u>Indications</u>: Non-depolarising neuromuscular blocker antagonist. Stimulates motility and tone of the GI tract. Miotic. Atropine poisoning/toxicity

  <u>Forms</u>: 2.5 mg/ml (1:500) aqueous injection in 1ml vials.

  <u>Dose</u>: 0.02 - 0.04 mg/kg IV/SC
  Dosing intervals determined by response.

  <u>Notes</u>: If overdose or muscarinic effects severe, treat with atropine (0.05mg/kg im). Magnesium may inhibit actions of anticholinesterase therapy.

h) Parasympatholytics

Atropine BP:
  Atrocare [*Animalcare Ltd*]
  Atropine Sulphate [*Boots*], [*Bimeda*], [*BK*] and [*VDC*].

  <u>Indications</u>: Parasympatholytic (anticholinegic, mydriatic, cycloplegic). Relief of smooth muscle spasm, antidote to parasympathomimetics (including organophosphates). For intraoperative bradydysrrythmias. In cardiopulmonary resuscitation. Bronchodilation.

  <u>Forms</u>: Clear aqueous solution, 10 mg/ml, 50 ml multidose vials.

  <u>Dose</u>: 0.04 - 0.06 mg/kg IV/IM/SC

  <u>Notes</u>: Side effects- (may be prolonged)
  Sinus tachycardia, ectopic complexes; vision disturbances, mydriasis, photophobia, cycloplegia, increased intra-occular pressure, (Mydriasis may cause panic - use darkened room); abdominal distension; ileus. Urinary retention.

i) Sympathomimetics

<u>**Dobutamine**</u>:   POM

Indications: Hypotension particularly during general anaesthesia. It is an inotropic agent indicated for short term support in patients with cardiac decompensation due to decreased contractility. Vascular effects are beleived to be minimal in other species. At normal doses cardiac rates are also not significantly affected, but rates may increase at higher dosages.

Forms: Dry powder 250 mg / bottle or 250 mg solution for dilution

Dose: Reconstitute with 1litre 5% glucose or 0.9% saline to yield a solution having a concentration of 250 ug/ml. Administer IV at 2 - 5 μg/kg/min

Notes: ECG monitoring for tachyarrhythmias essential.
Drug interactions: oxytocic drugs may cause a severe hypertension when used with dobutamine. Dobutamine may be ineffective if β blocking drugs eg. propanolol have recently been given.

<u>**Dopamine**</u>:   POM
Inotropin, Dopamine HCl in 5% Dextrose [*Abbott Labs*]*

Indications: Correction of haemodynamic imbalances in shock. Oliguric renal failure.

Forms:To prepare solution: add 250 mg to 1L of normal saline, D5W or Hartmans to give concentration of 250 μg/ml. * 250 ml flexible packs containing 200/400/800 μg/ml.

Dose: Variable according to effect desired (2 - 5 μg/kg/min) to promote urine output.
    5 - 10 μg/kg/min for β_1 effect.
    > 10 μg/kg/min causes α effect.

Notes: Only used in intensive care (esp neonates). Severe necrosis/sloughing if extravascular (if suspected infiltrate site with 5-10mg phentolamine in 10-15ml normal saline).
Monitor urine flow, cardiac rate/rhythm /blood pressure. In case of severe arrhythmias (PVC's) discontinue administration. Half life 5 - 9 minutes.

<u>**Ephedrine Sulphate**</u>:   POM

Indications: Indirect and direct pressor effects.

Forms: Aqueous solution for injection (50 mg/ml) 10 ml multidose vial.

Dose: 0.02-0.04mg/kg IV q 12h

Notes: VERY EXPENSIVE.

Epinephrine/Adrenaline: POM
Adrenaline 1-1000 [*Bimeda*]

Indications: Adrenergic (α and β). Bronchodilator. Increases systolic blood pressure. First line drug in cardiac resuscitation. Prolongs effect of local analgesics. Capillary haemostasis (local).

Forms: Clear, aqueous solution for injection. 1mg/ml (1 in 1000) as Adrenaline Acid Tartrate BP.

Doses: 0.1 - 0.2 ml/50kg by IV/IC injection.
0.2 - 0.4 ml/50kg by IM or SC injection.

Notes: Care with dose calculation. Best to dilute to 1 in 10000 using water for injection.

Isoprenaline: POM
Isuprel [*Winthrop Lab*]

Indications: Non-specific β receptor agonist. Emergency relief of bronchospasm. Has been used as positive inotrope.

Forms Injectable 1 in 5000 (0.2mg/ml) 1 ml vials

Dose: Best used as IV infusion administered to effect.

Notes: Causes dangerous tachycardia and arrythmias especially under halothane anaesthesia. Has been superseded by new specific β_1 agonist drugs.

Noradrenaline: POM
Levophed [*Winthrop)*

Indications: Predominantly α adrenergic effects (slight β effects).
For hypotension associated with anaesthesia.

Forms: 4mg in 4mls ampoules.

Dose: Dissolve 4mg in 1 litre saline solution. Administer as IV drip. Very short acting-administer according to effect.

Notes: Potent vasoconstrictor. May cause decreased organ perfusion and increased myocardial work. Avoid prolonged infusions.

Phenylephrine:
    Phenylephrine HCL [*Winthrop*]

    Indications: α adrenergic agonist. Useful in phenothiazine induced hypotension. May be used during anaesthesia.

    Forms: 1ml ampoules 10mg/ml

    Dose: 5 - 8 μg/kg IV will increase B.P. in Halothane anaesthetised horses.
    Most frequently used as a drip and administered to effect.

    Notes: High dose can increase myocardial work and decrease organ perfusion. Do not use in cases of myocardial failure.

j) Sympatholytics

Propanolol:
    Inderal [*ICI*]

    Indications: β-adrenoreceptor blocker (correction of supra-ventricular tachyarrhythmias).

    Forms: Aqueous injection (1 mg/ml) 1 ml glass vial.

    Dose: 0.05-0.15mg/kg IV slowly.

    Notes: Usually begin at low dose and titrate to effect. Can be used to correct serious tachydysrhythmias produced by β_1 agonists. NB drug is by definition a negative inotrope. Use with caution.

k) Opiate antagonists

Diprenorphine:
Revivon [*C-Vet Ltd*]

POM/CD (S-II)

<u>Indications</u>: Reversal of etorphine induced narcosis

<u>Forms</u>: Blue aqueous solution for injection 3 mg/ml, 10.5 ml multidose vial

<u>Dose</u>: Volume equal to the dose volume of etorphine used -IV. Further 50% may be given SC.

<u>Notes</u>: **NOT to be used for humans unless NO NARCAN available** (unforgivable circumstance!) (only use when clinical signs are seen). Initial dose for human is 0.1 ml IV/IM or preferably equal volume to the volume of etorphine injected. Repeat after 2 minutes IT IS, ITSELF, EXTREMELY UNPLEASANT when used in humans resulting in long term halucinations, dysphoria and nausea. You may wish that you <u>were</u> dead!

Naloxone:
Narcan [*Evans*]

POM/CD (S-II)

<u>Indications</u>: Respiratory depression associated with potent opiates.
Antidote against inadvertant human self administration of etorphine (L.A. Immobilon).

<u>Forms</u>: Single dose (1ml) vials 0.4 mg/ml for injection..

<u>Dose</u>: Adult- administer whole vial IM/<u>IV</u> injection. May need to repeat since half life is shorter (20 minutes) than etorphine.

<u>Notes</u>: **Call medical help immediately. Administer IV every 2 - 3 mins until symptoms are reversed and help arrives! If iv impossible use multi-site im injections**

l) Euthanasia solutions

Pentobarbitone Na: POM/CD (S-III)
  Euthatal [*RMB*]

  Indications: Euthenasia ONLY!

  Forms: Aqueous solution (200 mg/kg) for IV injection

  Dose: 1 ml / 3kg minimum.

  Notes: Use fast acting agent eg thiopentone Na first or mixed with solution. Induction may be slow and accompanied by significant and distressing excitement.

Quinalbarbitone Sodium BP: POM/CD (S-II)
  Somulose (with Cinchocaine HCl)) [*Arnolds*]

  Indications: Euthenasia ONLY!

  Forms: Thick aqueous solution (400 mg/kg) for IV injection

  Dose: 1 ml / 20kg minimum. Ponies - 15ml, Horses 25-35 ml

  Notes: SPEED OF INJECTION IMPORTANT - too fast gives excitement, too slow prolonged anaesthesia! Best to use 16 g catheter - injection should take 10-15 secs. Keep adequate restraint until collapse - normally 30-45 secs (Longer if premedicated with Detomidine/Xylazine etc). Death usually rapid after gentle collapse.

NOTES

NOTES

NOTES

SECTION 2: *CARDIO-VASCULAR AGENTS:*

a) Anti-arrhythmic drugs:

Propanolol: See p53

Quinidine Sulphate: Not applicable
Analytical Reagent [*Sigma*]

Indications: Treatment of supraventricular cardiac arrhythmias (particularly atrial fibrillation, premature ventricular beats and ventricular tachycardia).

Presentation: Powder for oral administration

Dose: 10 mg /kg PO q 2 h until effects seen. Maximum total dose 80 mg/kg in any 24 hour period.

NORMAL REGIME: for 500 kg horse: Day 1: test dose (5 g) (by stomach tube in solution). If safe proceed to Day 2: 10 gram doses (po) at 2 hour intervals. Careful cardiac monitoring (ECG). Continue until conversion or up to 8th dose (ie total 80 grams). If not converted wait until next day and start again. If reverts or no conversion then may need persistent treatment using 10 g q12h on day 1 & 2, 10 g q8h days 3 & 4, 10 g q6h days 5 & 6, 15 g q6h days 7 & 8. If converted use half dose for next 24 hours. Then cease.

Notes: TEST DOSE of 5 mg/kg (5 grams) given to detect untoward effects (nasal congestion, laryngeal and pulmonary oedema, urticaria, laminitis, colic, diarrhoea, cardiac arrythmia). Early indications of toxicity by > 75% lengthening of QRS complex on ECG.
If congestive heart failure (CHF) present digitalise first (qv). If no CHF is present DO NOT digitalise. Risk of death!
Toxic to humans - absorbed through skin! Wear gloves.

b) Cardiac glycosides:

Digoxin: POM
   Lanoxin [*Welcome*]

   Indications: Congestive heart failure, supraventricular arrhythmias

   Presentation: 0.25 mg tabs
            0.25 mg /ml injection in 2 ml single dose vials

   Dose: 0.06 - 0.08 mg/kg PO q 8h increased by 50% every 2nd day to effect

   Notes: Horses with CHF should be digitalised before administration of Quinidine Sulphate (but those with no CHF should NOT) although the two drugs should not be given simultaneously. Side effects include sudden death, A-V block, arrhythmias, anorexia, diarrhoea, depression. Blood levels should be monitored carefully, particularly if no effects are seen.

c) Anticholinergics:

Atropine Sulphate: see p50

Glycopyrrolate: POM
   Robinul [*Wellcome*]

   Indications: Anticholinergic

   Forms: Aqueous injection (0.2 mg/ml)

   Dose: 5 - 10 μg/kg IV

   Notes: More expensive than atropine. Supposedly more potent anti-sialagogue with fewer arrythmogenic tendencies. Advantage over atropine in the horse has not been proven.

d) Vasodilating agents

Isoxuprine: POM

Duviculin [*Duphar*], Navilox [*Univet*], Oralject Circulon [*Millpledge*]

<u>Indications</u>: Vasodilator of peripheral capillaries esp. in skeletal muscle. Indicated in treatment of Navicular Disease and myo-ischaemia/myopathies

<u>Forms</u>: 20 mg tablets Oral, 60 mg palatable capsules for oral dosing.
230 ml (40mg/ml) solution for oral dosing

<u>Dose</u>: 0.6 - 0.7 mg/kg PO q12h for 21 days then q 24h for 7 days, then alternate days.

<u>Notes</u>: High doses may impair platelet aggregation and reduce blood viscosity. NOT FOR PREGNANT MARES or where haemorrhagic disorders have been identified.

e) Shock treatments:

Epinephrine/Adrenaline: p52

Dobutamine: p51

Dopamine:p51

See also: **FLUID THERAPY (p131)**
            CORTICOSTEROIDS (p93)

NOTES

SECTION 3: *RESPIRATORY DRUGS:*

NOTES

a) Bronchodilators:

Clenbuterol: POM
Ventipulmin [*Boehringer Ingelheim*]

Indications: Sympathomimetic (adrenergic). Bronchodilator (COPD); acute, subacute or chronic allergic bronchitis with bronchospasm. Adjuvant therapy for respiratory infections (virus and bacterial)

Forms: Powder for oral feed administration 0.016 mg/g
Syrup for oral dosing/in feed 25μg/ml in dispensing pump.
Aqueous solution for injection 0.03 μg/ml

Dose: 0.8μg/kg po q 12h (1 level measure / 200 kg)
0.8 μg/kg IV/IM (1.25 ml / 50kg)

Notes: Parenteral dose effective for 12 hours (useful initially followed by oral q 12h). Antagonises effects of $PGF_2\alpha$ and oxytocin. Discontinue at expected delivery time. May reduce unwanted uterine contractions (higher dose regime).

Etamphyline camsylate: POM
Millophyline [*Arnolds*]

Indications: Pneumonia / upper respiratory tract infections (supportive). Cardiovascular collapse or respiratory failure. Pleuritis, Pulmonary oedema and syncope.

Forms: Aqueous solution 140 mg/ml for injection IM/SC
White soluble powder 300 mg single dose sachet po.

Dose: 20 - 30 mg/kg IM/SC q 8-24 h OR 3 sachets q 8h po

Notes: Side effect includes CNS stimulation. IV slow/diluted.

68

Theophyline:
Euphyllin(with Euphyllin)[*Boehringer Ingelheim*]

Indications: Spasmolytic - relief of bronchospasm and pulmonary oedema. Supportive therapy for COPD-Small Airway Disease. Mild diuretic.

Forms: 20 ml multidose vial 25 mg/ml for IV injection
3 g (with 3.67 g Euphyllin) individual dose sachets

Dose: 12 mg/kg IV initial dose then 6 mg/kg IV q12h
Powder for oral in-feed use.

Notes: Dilute in saline before injection and administer slowly. IM causes marked pain. Excitement, tremors, visual disturbances, ataxia may be seen. Antagonistic effect with B blockers eg propanolol. Do not administer to animals with myocardial disease or pregnant mares.

b) Antihistamines

<u>Sodium Cromoglycate</u>:   POM
    Cromovet [*Fisons*]

    <u>Indications</u>: Prophylaxis and control of respiratory tract allergic conditions/COPD

    <u>Presentation</u>: 4 ml glass/plastic ampoules 80 mg Sodium Cromoglycate.

    <u>Dose</u>: Single ampoule administered via nebuliser (mask), q24h for 4 days.

    <u>Notes</u>: Single courses expected to provide prophylaxis for 3 - 20 days (Not predictable). MUST
    be accompanied by full range of management / supportive measures.
    Do not administer in first trimester of pregnancy.

<u>Tripelanamine</u>:   POM
    Bimahistamine [*Bimeda*], Vetibenzamine [*Ciba-Geigy*],
    Salophen Co (with dexamethasone and chloramphenicol [*Arnolds*])

    <u>Indications</u>: Acute allergic, anaphylactic and sensitivity reactions including urticaria and
    photosensitisation.

    <u>Forms</u>: Parenteral solution for IV or IM injection 20 mg/ml multidose vials (100 ml)

    <u>Dose</u>: O.5 mg per kg q8h IV/IM (240mg max dose)

    <u>Notes</u>: Not to be administered to animals incapable of locomotion eg fractures. Particular care
    with young animals.
    Estimate body weight accurately. Do not administer SC.

c) Antitussives

Butorphenol Tartrate: see Analgesics (p39)

Codeine Phosphate BP: POM/CD (S-V)

    Indications: Diarrhoea, cough suppression

    Forms: Tablets 60mg.

    Dose: 0.2-2g/day.

    Notes: Symptomatic treatment only.

Diphenhydramine: POM
  Benylin [*Parke Davis*]

    Indications: Suppression of coughing

    Forms: Syrup for oral dosing

    Dose: 25 - 30 ml PO q8h

    Notes: Mild sedation may follow. Do not use if animal to be ridden.

d) Mucolytics:

Bromhexine HCl: POM
Bisolvon [*Boehringer Ingelheim*],

Indications: Assists control and treatment of respiratory tract infections and hypersensitivity conditions eg COPD.

Presentation: Oral powder (10 mg/g)
                Aqueous solution for injection (3 mg/ml)

Dose: 0.1 - 0.3 mg /kg oral/parenteral daily for up to 5 days or longer. 1.5 mg /kg IM/IV q 12h.

Notes: Parenteral dose may be useful initially followed by oral use. May safely be administered over prolonged courses. Contra-indications minimal.
May be mixed with sulphonamides/potentiated sulphonamides for oral use (Clenbuterol/TMP/S

Dembrexine: POM
Sputolosin [*Boehringer Ingelheim*]

Indications: Symptomatic treatment of acute or chronic respiratory disease.

Presentation: Powder 5 mg/gram active ingredient. Multidose 420 gram tub. (Measure enclosed)

Dose: 0.3 mg /kg in feed q12h for 12 - 14 days.

Notes: Very safe. Do not exceed 28 days treatment (reassess case). Concurrent antibiotics may be indicated. May be mixed with sulphonamides/potentiated sulphonamides and/or clenbuterol for oral use.
Not for use in pregnant mares.

NOTES

SECTION 4: *URINARY TRACT DRUGS:*

NOTES

a) Diuretics

Furosemide:
    Lasix [*Hoechst*]

<u>Indications</u>: Oedematous conditions, congestive heart failure, allergic oedema, supportive therapy in laminitis and renal failure, paralytic myoglobinuria.
Exercise Induced Pulmonary Haemorrhage

<u>Presentation</u>: Aqueous 5 % solution for injection (50 mg/ml), 10 ml multidose vial

<u>Dose</u>: 0.5-1.0 mg/kg IV/IM q12-24h pnr.

<u>Notes</u>: Potent saluretic diuretic. Rapid onset (increased Na^+ / water excretion without significant loss of K^+ over short courses). Severe conditions may require double dosage.
Monitor electrolytes over treatment course.
DO NOT use if glomerulonephritis, renal failure with anuria and electrolyte deficiency syndromes present. Restrict water intake during treatment.
Effects on Exercise Induced Pulmonary Haemorrhage limited (Probably does not reduce haemorrhage).

Hydrochlorothiazide:
    Vetidrex [*Ciba Geigy*]

<u>Indications</u>: Chronic/pathological oedema, insect bites, sheath swellings etc.

<u>Presentation</u>: Aqueous sol. 50 mg/ml for injection (10 ml multidose vials)
             Dispersable tablets (250 mg) for oral administration

<u>Dose</u>: 0.5 mg/kg IM/IV q24h prn
      1.0 mg/kg PO as drench or in feed.

<u>Notes</u>: Warm solution to blood heat when IV. Increases K^+ excretion and sensitises myocardium to digitalis. Consider potassium supplementation.

Mannitol:

Indications: Osmotic diuresis, reduction of intracranial (CSF) and intra-ocular pressure. Aids excretion of endotoxins.

Forms: 25% solution for injection in 50 ml single dose vial.

Dose: 0.25 - 2.0 g/kg slow IV (drip)

Notes: Increases Na^+, K^+ and Cl^- loss. Check for crystals (warm solution). Do not use in CHF, pulmonary oedema, anuric renal failure. Monitor electrolytes. Do NOT mix with other electrolyte solutions unless very diluted (precipitates)!

NOTES

NOTES

SECTION 5: *GASTROINTESTINAL AGENTS:*

a) Antacids/Anti-Ulcer drugs:

Cimetidine: POM
> Tagamet [*Pitman-Moore*]

> Indications: Histamine (H_2) receptor antagonist. Used to treat/prevent gastric and duodenal ulcers. Adjunct therapy for metabolic alkalosis.

> Presentation: 300mg tablet for oral use
>> 100 mg/ml solution for injection (2 ml single dose vials)

> Dose: 8 - 10 mg /kg IV q 8-12h
>> 24 mg /kg PO q 12h

> Notes: Poor gut absorbtion so higher oral doses. Reduces hepatic clearance of warfarin, B blockers, quinidine sulphate, metronidazole, diazepam. Stagger dose (2 hrs) when used with sucralfate.

Ranitidine: POM
> Zantac [*Pitman-Moore*]

> Indications: As for **Cimetidine** (above)

> Presentation: 150 mg tablet oral
>> Solution for injection, ?5mg/ml.

> Dose: 6 mg/kg PO q12-24h
>> 3 mg/kg IV q 24h

> Notes: More expensive than cimetidine but less frequent dosing necessary.

Sucralfate: POM
> Antepsin [*Ayerst Labs*]

> Indications: Gastro-intestinal ulceration. In acid medium forms non-absorbable ion (binds to protein exudates creating "bandage" over ulcers).

> Forms: 1 gr tablet, Oral

> Dose: Foals 2 grams PO q6 - 8h
>> Adults 2 - 4 grams PO q6 - 8h

> Notes: Should be given on empty stomach (> 1 hour before feed) Availability of H_2 blockers (qv) may be impaired if given at same time. Also requires acid environment so do not give at same time as H_2 blockers or antacids (not strictly necessary). Drug is complex of aluminium hydroxide and sulphated sucrose.

b) Intestinal stimulants:

Cisapride:

Cisapride [*Janssen*]

Indications: Prophylaxis/treatment of ileus.

Forms: Solution for injection 5mg/ml.

Dose: 0.1mg/kg IM (3, 11 and 19 hours post operatively, q 8h until motility returns.

Notes: G-I prokinetic with cholinergic action. Possible role in the treatment of pelvic flexure impactions and gastric ulceration. NOT READILY AVAILABLE/SOON TO BE UNAVAILABLE.

c) Intestinal sedatives:

Hyoscine-n-butyl bromide:

Buscopan Compositum (with Dipyrone)[*Boehringer Ingelheim*]

Indications: Intestinal antispasmodic - treatment of spasmodic colic and obstructive colic and aids rectal examination. Aids relief of oesophageal intra-luminal obstructions.

Forms: Sterile aqueous solution for injection, 100 ml multidose vials (4 mg /ml hyoscine + 500 mg/ml dipyrone).

Dose: 0.5 mg/kg IV (20-30ml).

Notes: Dipyrone is non-steroidal analgesic. Failure of colic to respond may indicate more severe problems (investigate further). NOT FOR IM injection (marked local reaction). Extravascular injection may cause thrombophlebitis.

d) Laxatives/Cathartics

Danthrone (Dihydroxyanthraquinone)   POM
    Altan [*May Baker*], Physic Powder,

    Indications: Purgative,laxative.

    Presentation: Insoluble powder for suspension in water.
    Dose: 15-30g/450kg

    Notes: Acts on large and small colon after absorbtion and metabolisation. Effects are often severe. Do not exceed dose.

Dioctyl Sodium Sulfosuccinate: PML
    Surfactol [*Centaur*]

    Indications: Intestinal impactions, fermentative colic.

    Forms: Water and oil based solution for oral use only

    Dose: Up to 0.2g/kg by stomach tube.

    Notes: Surfactant laxative. Not recommended for use with liquid paraffin.

Liquid paraffin BP: GSL

    Indications: Impactions of the intestines,particularly pelvic flexure impactions.

    Forms: Oily liquid

    Dose: 2-6 litres by stomach tube/pump

    Notes: Administration facilitated by mixing with warm water.
    Not practical to dose effective amounts by drenching.

Magnesium Sulphate BP: GSL
    Epsom Salt [*Univet*]

    Indications: Intestinal impactions.

    Forms: Crystals/powder (100%).

    Dose: 100-400g/450kg.

    Notes: Osmotic laxative. Effects often severe.

Sodium Phosphate/biphosphate enema: POM
   [*Bimeda*]

Indications: Meconium retention,small colon/rectal impactions.

Forms: Suppositories or plastic packs with extension nozzle.

Dose: pnr

Notes: Safe, reliable, effective. Multiple enemas (of any type) may cause mucosal irritation /
oedema.

Sodium Sulphate BP: GSL/P
   Glaubers Salt [*BDH*]

Indications: Intestinal impactions,purgation.

Presentation: Crystals/powder.

Dose: 100–400g/450kg.

Notes: Very safe.

e) Antidiarrheals:

Codeine Phosphate BP: POM/CD (S-V)

Indications: Diarrhoea, cough suppression

Forms: Tablets 60mg.

Dose: 0.2 - 2g/day.

Notes: Symptomatic treatment only.

NOTES

NOTES

SECTION 6: HORMONES:

a) Prostaglandins

NB: Absorbed through human skin. Should not be handled by women of child bearing age. Accidental skin contact should be washed immediately with cold water. May also cause bronchospasm. DO NOT USE WITH NON-STEROIDAL ANTI-INFLAMMATORY DRUGS

<u>Alfaprostol</u>:   POM
    Alphacept [*Beecham*]

<u>Indications</u>: Luteolytic control of oestrous cycle (including termination of persistent dioestrus, control of sub-oestrus and induction of abortion. Treatment of prolonged dioestrus

<u>Forms</u>: Sterile aqueous solution for injection, 40 ml multidose vials 2mg/ml

<u>Dose</u>: 2 - 10 mg **total dose IM**

<u>Notes</u>: Sweating, abdominal discomfort, tachycardia, polypnea. Spontaneous resolution after 5 - 10 mins.

<u>Cloprostenol</u>:   POM
    Estrumate [*Coopers*]

<u>Indications</u>: Luteolytic control of oestrous cycle (including termination of persistent dioestrus, control of sub-oestrus and induction of abortion. Treatment of prolonged dioestrus

<u>Forms</u>: Sterile aqueous solution for injection, 10 ml multidose vials 250 μg/ml IM

<u>Dose</u>: 125 - 250 μg **total dose IM**

<u>Notes</u>: Sweating, abdominal discomfort, tachycardia, polypnea. Spontaneous resolution after 5 - 10 mins.

<u>Dinoprost promethamine</u>:   POM
    Lutalyse [*Upjohn*]

<u>Indications</u>: Luteolytic control of oestrus cycle, treatment of sub-oestrus, abortion induction (at certain stages)(including termination of persistent dioestrus, control of sub-oestrus. Treatment of prolonged dioestrus

<u>Forms</u>: Aqueous solution for injection 5 mg/ml

<u>Dose</u>: 5 mg **total dose IM**

<u>Notes</u>: Side effects include sweating, colic (usually disappear spontaneously after 10 - 15 mins).

b) Sex steroid hormones

Allyl Trenbolone:
Regumate [*Hoechst*]

Indications: Induction of cyclic ovarian activity either early in the season or in response to poor cyclicity at other stages.
Treatment of lactation anoestrus in absence of corpus luteum.
Suppression of oestrus and oestrous behaviour. Managemental manipulation of oestrus cycle.

Forms: Vegetable oil solution for oral use 2.2 mg/ml, multidose container with dose regulating cup built in.

Dose: +ve ovarian activity: 12 ml q 24 h for 10 consecutive days
      -ve ovarian activity: 12 ml q 24 h for 10 days
      Courses of 15 days or more may be used to suppress or regulate oestrus.

Notes: Do not use in pregnant mares / stallions. Recommended by W.R. Allen for treatment of habitual aborters. Not for horses for human consumption. Mixing with feed should be immediately before administration.
Women of child bearing age should not handle the product. Protective measures (gloves, sleeves etc) should be used when handling concentrate or feed.

Oestradiol Benzoate: POM
Oestradiol Benzoate [*Intervet*]

Indications:Short term oestrogen therapy. Sub-oestrus.

Forms: Oily solution for injection 5mg/ml multidose vial.

Dose: 10 -15 mg single **total dose IM**

Notes: Virilising or excessive oestrus effects may be seen.
       USE WITH CAUTION

Testosterone :   POM
    Androject [*Intervet*], Durateson [*Intervet*], Testosterone implants [*Intervet*]

    <u>Indications</u>: Long term androgen therapy (up to 60 days). Ageing and debility. Possible improved libido in stallion.

    <u>Forms</u>: Oily solution for injection 10 mg/ml 10 ml multidose vial
          Solid 25 mg single tablet for subcutaneous deposition

    <u>Dose</u>: 300 - 500 mg **total dose**

    <u>Notes</u>: Virilism may occur. Purpose made trochar and canula is useful.
    USE WITH EXTREME CAUTION - long courses probably detrimental to spermatogenesis.

Pregnant Mare Serum Gonadotrophin [FSH]:   POM
    Prostim [*Upjohn*], Folligon [*Upjohn*], Fostim [*Paines and Bryne*]

    <u>Indications</u>: PROBABLY NO EFFECT IN MARES

Human Chorionic Gonadotrophin [Luteinising Hormone]:   POM
    Chorulon [*Intervet*], Nymphalon (with progesterone)[*Intervet*]

    <u>Indications</u>: Stimulation of ovulation, formation of corpus luteum.
    Suboestrus (follicles >2cm), Post-partum lactation failure, nymphomania, prolonged oestrus.
    Used as part of test for cryptorchidism (page 19). Poor libido in stallions

    <u>Forms</u>: Single dose vials, 1500 iu, white soluble powder. Solvent supplied.

    <u>Dose</u>: 1,500 - 3,000 iu IV prn

    <u>Notes</u>: IM/SC injections may abscessate/clostridial myositis. Rare anaphylaxis after IV.
        When used for lactational failure oxytocin (qv) should be given simultaneously

Progesterone: POM
   Progesterone Implant [*Intervet*], Progesterone Injection [*Intervet*]

   Indications: Habitual abortion

   Forms: Sterile solid tablets 50 / 100 mg for subcutaneous deposition using trochar and cannula
   supplied.
         Sterile oily solution 25 mg /ml for injection

   Dose: 100 mg daily IM
         800 mg total dose (1st trimester) SC implant
         600 mg total dose (2nd/3rd trimester) SC implant

   Notes: Disputed efficacy in maintaining effective elevation in blood progesterone. 100 mg
   implants suggested to have 250 day effect. 50 mg implant lasts 200 days.
   Implants should be removed at specified time to avoid prolongation of pregnancy.

Buserelin: POM
   Receptal [*Hoechst*]

   Indications: Infertility of ovarian origin. Improvement of conception rates.

   Forms: Aqueous solution for injection 0.004 mg/ml

   Dose: 10 ml total dose single IV,IM or SC injection, administered on first day of maximum
   follicle size, 6 hours before service. Repeat 24 hours if ovulation not taken place.

   Notes: Synthetic Gn-RH analogue.

c) Anabolic steroids:

Boldenone Undecyclenate: POM
Vebonol [*Ciba-Geigy*]

Indications: Anabolic stimulation, metabolic enhancement

Forms: 25 mg/ml in oily solution for IM injection

Dose: 2.0 mg/kg IM. Repeated at 2 - 3 week intervals

Notes: Administration to geldings at full dose may induce masculine behaviour (use half dose at 10 day intervals). Contraindicated in all neoplastic conditions.

d) Posterior pituitary hormones:

Oxytocin: POM
Oxytocin-S [*Intervet*], Pituitary Injection (BVet C) [*Arnolds*](Natural extract),
Pituitary Injection (BVet C) [*Pharmavet*](Natural extract),
Pituitary Injection (BVet C) [*Univet*](Natural extract),
Pituitary Extract (BVet C) [*Animalcare Ltd*],

Indications: Stimulation of smooth muscle in uterus and mammary gland. Induction of parturition. Treatment of retained placenta.

Forms: Sterile aqueous solution for injection 10 iu/ml multidose 25 ml vial

Dose: 25-100 iu SC/IM. 50 iu in 250 ml saline as IV infusion for placental retention.
2 - 10 iu IV for parturition induction.

Notes: Sweating, colic may be seen. ONLY to be used for induction of parturition when milk calcium concentration $\geq$ 10 mmol/l.

e) Adrenal corticoids:

Corticosteroids are potentially very dangerous in inducing or exacerbating laminitis and are specifically CONTRAINDICATED IN THE TREATMENT OF LAMINITIS and related conditions. The clinician is warned that due deliberation should be given before any horse is subjected to systemic or oral corticosteroid therapy.

<u>Betamethasone</u>:   POM
    Betsolan [*Pitman-Moore*], Betsolan/Betnesol/Vetsovate Oph/ear Drops[*Pitman-Moore*],
    Vetsovate/Betsolan Ointment [*Pitman-Moore*]

<u>Indications</u>: Shock, inflammatory and hypersensitivity reactions/pruritis. Arthritis

<u>Forms</u>: β-Na Phosphate true solution 2mg/ml for IV.
       β- suspension 2mg/ml for IM.

<u>Dose</u>: 0.1 - 0.3 mg /kg IV/IM (Check formulation)

<u>Notes</u>: Do not use suspension IV. Interactions/precautions as for Dexamethasone (below).
Contraindicated as part of topical or systemic therapy where infectious agent are involved and
where corneal ulcers are present.

<u>Dexamethasone</u>:   POM
    Azium (*) [*Schering-Plough*], Soludex [*Mycofarm*]
    Dexadreson [*Intervet*], Adzoid [*Arnolds*], Dexazone[*Bimeda*],
    Voren (1 mg/ml Dexamethasone-21-isonicotinate)[*Boehringer Ingelheim*],
    Voren 14 (3mg/ml Dexamethasone-21-isonicotinate)[*Boehringer Ingelheim*],
    Streptovin [*Pitman-Moore*, with penicillin/streptomycin],
    Opticorten Tablets (with prednisolone) [*Ciba-Geigy*], Oticortenol-S [*Ciba-Geigy*],
    Duphacort [*Duphar*], Diodex [*Alan Hitchins*],
    Dexafort [*Intervet*], Duocort [*Norbrook*], Panasone [*Norbrook*],
    (* as dexamethasone alcohol)

<u>Indications</u>: Treatment of inflamatory/hypersensitivity conditions. Specifically Treatment of
Purpura Haemorrhagica. Azoturia. Immune suppression

<u>Forms</u>: Systemic: 2 mg /ml Dexamethasone Na phosphate in aqueous or alcoholic solution. Most
in 50 ml multidose vials.
Oral: 5mg tablet (Opticorten)

<u>Dose</u>: 0.1 - 2.0 mg /kg IV/IM (Higher doses for shock and hypersensitivity conditions, lower
dose range for inflamatory conditions)

<u>Notes</u>: * Alcoholic form physiologically available immediately.
Possible reactivation of latent Herpes Virus. Drug interactions with Amphoteracin B, K^+
depleting diuretics eg furosemide, thiazides. May increase urine glucose and decrease T_3 and T_4
concentrations. Dexamethasone-21-isonicotinate (*3mg/ml) reported to have 7 - 14 day activity.
CHECK FORMULATION BEFORE INJECTION -CONFIRM ROUTE COMPATIBILITY

Fluomethasone: POM
Fluvet 50 Injection [*Syntex*], Fluvet (with DMSO)[*Syntex*],

Indications: Myositis, dermatoses, allergies, inflammatory conditions

Forms: Sterile aqueous solution for injection 0.5 mg/ml 50 ml multidose vial

Dose: 0.05 mg/kg q 24 h IV/IM prn

Notes: See notes for corticosteroids above.

Methylprednisolone:
Depomedrone [*Upjohn*], Solumedrone [*Upjohn*]

Indications: Shock, anti-inflammatory therapy, immune supression.

Forms: M~- acetate (Depomedrone) insoluble ester for IM injection in 5 ml vials; M~-sodium succinate (Solumedrone) soluble ester for IV injection in Mix-o-vials of 125 mg and 500 mg.

Dose: 0.2 - 0.7 mg/kg IM (>10x this dose for shock!)

Notes: Soluble form IV for rapid effect.

Prednisolone: POM
Flamasone [*Norbrook*], Prednivet [*Willows Francis*], Depomedrone [*Upjohn*]
Opticorten (with dexamethasone)[*Ciba-Geigy*], Opticortenol-S (with dexamethasone)[*Ciba-Geigy*]

Indications: Anti-inflammatory, anti-allergic parenteral therapy. Anorexia following overtraining, shipping or unusual physical exertion. Immune supression. Temporary treatment of malabsorbtion/intestinal lymphosarcoma

Forms: Injectable: Pred-Na Succinate 500 mg/ml (usually 5/10 ml   multidose vials)
10 mg/ml aqueous suspension (20 - 50 ml multidose vials)
5 mg tablet (oblet) for oral dosing
Ophthalmic: Pred- acetate 1% Ophth Sol.

Dose: Prednisolone acetate injection: 0.25 -1.0 mg/kg IM;
40 - 80 mg intra-articular (CARE).
Oral: 0.2 - 0.5 mg/kg

Notes: Sodium succinate should be used for immediate effects. Interactions as for dexamethasone (qv).
Intra-articular injection rarely indicated (frequently followed by infections) (scrupulous asepsis)..
Prolonged courses should be terminated gradually (3 - 5 days).

Triamcinolone: POM
   Vetalog [*Ciba-Geigy*]

Indications: Dermatoses, inflammatory conditions

Forms: Suspension 6 mg/ml triamcinolone acetonide

Dose: 0.02 - 0.1 mg/kg IM

Notes: See general note for corticosteroids above. SERIOUS RISK OF LAMINITIS.

f) Non-steroidal anti-inflamatory drugs:

Acetylsalycilic acid: POM
Aspirin BP, Tensolvet* [C-Vet]

Indications: Antipyretic, analgesic, anti-inflammatory

Forms: 325 mg tablet
White powder
* Topical solution

Dose: 100 mg/kg q 8h PO
* Topical applied to shaved/clipped skin q 12h prn

Notes: Platelet aggregation (and bleeding times) may be affected

Dimethylsulphoxide: POM

Demavet[Syntex], Fluvet DMSO (with flumethasone) [Syntex]

Indications: Topical/IV anti-inflammatory. Decreases intracranial pressure. Used as carrier - aids skin penetration of other drugs eg corticosteroids.

Forms: 90% solution in non sterile analytical reagent bottles. Premixed in bottles with steroids for topical application to skin (applicator or paint brush supplied)

Dose: 0.25 - 1 .0 g/kg very slow IV as diluted (20%) solution in Normal saline. High doses to control intra cranial pressure (110 mls in 1 1 saline as drip for 500kg horse).
Topical: apply 3 - 4 times daily to shaved area

Notes: Handle with care. Rapid skin penetration. Wear gloves. May show diuretic effect when given IV. If given fast may cause significant haemolysis.

Dipyrone: POM
Buscopan Compositum (with hyoscine)[Boehringer Ingelheim]

Indications: Pyrazoline analgesic, antipyretic, anti-inflammatory

Forms: Multidose vials most often with other drugs in mixtures.

Dose: 22 mg/kg IV

Notes: Do not use with phenothiazine ataractics (hypothermia). May cause blood dyscrasias, hepatitis, nephropathy, colic, diarrhoea. DO NOT OVERDOSE. NOT IM.

Flunixin meglumine: POM
  Finadyne [*Schering Plough*].

  Indications: Analgesia, antipyresis, Strong anti-inflammatory effect. Strong anti-endotoxin effects.

  Forms: Solution for injection (50 mg/ml) 50 ml multidose vials.
    Sachets (10g) containing 250mg flunixin for oral administration
    Paste (10g) containing 500mg flunixin for oral dosing

  Dose: 1.1 mg/kg IV or IM q24h
      1.1 mg/kg oral q24h
      0.25 - 0.55 mg/kg q8h for endotoxaemia

  Notes: NOT used with other NSAIDs (toxic effects additive). Use with great care in colic (masks
  signs indicating surgical condition - risk of visceral rupture before surgery).
  Anti-endotoxin effects best at 0.25 - 0.55 mg/kg q12h/q8h.

Isopyrin: POM
  Tomanol (with phenylbutazone) [*Intervet*]

  Indications: Analgesia, antipyresis, anti-inflammatory effect.

  Forms: Solution 240 mg isopyrin and 130 mg phenylbutazone sodium /ml.

  Dose: 4.2 mg/kg phenylbutazone and 7.8 mg/kg isopyrin IV q24h.

  Notes: The dose dependent kinetics of phenylbutazone mean that its half-life is extended by
  mixing with another pyrazolone. This explains the recommendation for daily dosing only.

Meclofenamic Acid: POM
  Arquel [*Parke Davis*], Equafen [*Duphar*]

  Indications: Anti-inflammatory, analgesic, antipyretic

  Forms: 10 g sachets for oral use in feed.

  Dose: 2.2 mg/kg q24h.

  Notes: Manufacturers only advise continuing treatment for maximum of seven days.

Naproxen: POM
    Equiproxen Granules [*Syntex*]

    Indications: Relief of inflammation and pain associated with muscle and soft tissues. Marked
    analgesic and antipyretic effects. (Prostaglandin inhibitor)

    Forms: Single dose sachets (4 grams active substance in granule form) for oral use.

    Dose: 10 mg/kg po q 12 h in feed for 14 days (pnr)

    Notes: Not to be used in pregnancy. Safe.

Phenylbutazone: POM
    Equipalazone [*Arnolds*], Intrazone [*Arnolds*], Butaleucotropin (with cinchopen) [*Berk*],
    Phenyzene [*C-Vet*], Tomanol (with isopyrin)[*Intervet*]

    Indications: Analgesia, antipyresis

    Forms: Oral, white powder / individual sachets (1 g, 0.5 g) or oral paste in dose graduated (kg)
    syringe; Parenteral: solution 200mg/ml (Tomanol see isopyrin).

    Dose: Solution: 4.4 mg/kg IV.
        Oral: DAY1: 4.4 mg/kg q12h, 2.2 mg/kg q12h days 2-5, then 2.2 mg/kg q24h or
        q48h pnr

    Notes: Do not use IM. As with all NSAIDs (excluding aspirin), phenylbutazone strongly protein
    bound. Therefore care should be exercised if concurrent use with other protein bound agents.

g) Others

Adrenocorticotrophic Hormone: POM
   Cortrosyn [*Organon, USA*], Synacthen [*Ciba Labs*]

   Indications: Stimulation of adrenal activity in premature/dysmature foals. Diagnosis of pituitary-adrenal axis disorders.

   Presentation: 1ml single use vials or 2 ml multidose vials (250ug/ml).

   Dose: 0.4 mg total dose for 50 kg foal IM, q 12 h rep 3 days

   Notes: Single doses may be effective in foals. Long acting form available as Synacthen Depot (1mg/ml in 1ml vials or 2ml multidose vials). Long acting (gel) form may be used to identify primary or secondary adrenocortical deficiency.

Insulin PTZ: POM
   Insulin PTZ [*Boots*]

   Indications: Specific therapy for insulin responsive Diabetes mellitus. Treatment of Hyperlipaemia in ponies

   Forms: Granular aqueous suspension 40 / 100 iu /ml 10 ml multidose vial

   Dose: Titration in diabetes mellitus. Lipaemia: 40 iu IM q 24 h.

   Notes: Treatment of Lipaemia should be carried out with oral (or iv) glucose therapy at 0.25g /kg po q 12 h.

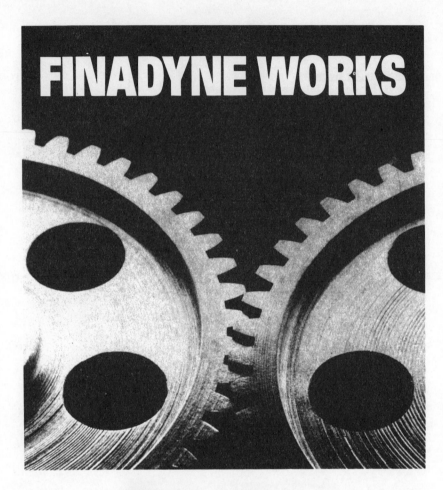

FINADYNE WORKS

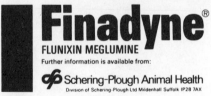

Finadyne®

FLUNIXIN MEGLUMINE

Further information is available from:

SECTION 7: *ANTI-INFECTIVE DRUGS:*

Telmin

The wormer
that's powerful enough for hunters
yet gentle enough for foals

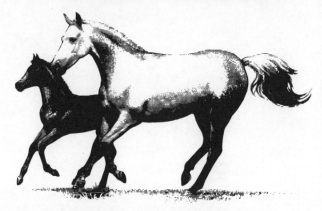

Because horses usually represent a substantial investment in both financial and emotional terms, regular worming is extremely important.

Telmin* is a powerful wormer which can be used to treat all types of horses and ponies. However, due to its gentle action, Telmin* is particularly suitable for brood mares and young foals. It is available as granules, or as a smooth paste in a syringe.

Telmin* is on sale at saddlers, agricultural merchants or from your vet.

Telmin
TRADEMARK

Kills worms
with gentle power

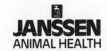

JANSSEN
ANIMAL HEALTH

TURNING RESEARCH INTO REALITY

Further information is available from:
Janssen Animal Health, Janssen Pharmaceutical Ltd,
Grove, Wantage, Oxon OX12 0DQ Tel: (0235) 772966

Product Information: Telmin* granules contain 2g mebendazole per sachet. Telmin* paste contains 4g mebendazole per syringe. Not to be used in animals intended for slaughter for human consumption. © JAH/031/92

a) Anthelmintics:

* Note regular worm egg counts should be used to monitor the effects of anthelmintic programs and the occurrence of resistance. Routine worming programs should be adjusted to suit the circumstances and the efficiency of clean pasture management. Full therapeutic doses should be used at all times.

<u>Dichlorvos</u>:   POM
Astrobot [*Arnolds*]

<u>Indications</u>: Control and removal of large and small strongyles, bots and oxyuris, ascarids.

<u>Forms</u>: Granules in single dose sachets

<u>Dose</u>: 1 sachet / 250 kg bodyweight

<u>Notes</u>: Organophosphate toxicity possible. Dispose of dung carefully - very toxic to fish and chickens. Occasional severe reactions follow sudden kill of heavy burdens.

<u>Fenbendazole</u>:   PML
Panacur [*Hoechst*]

<u>Indications</u>: Anthelmintic treatment and control programs for all types of helminth parasites of horses.

<u>Forms</u>: Paste in dosing syringe (graduated kg),
    10g sachets (granules[22%]) for in-feed administration,
    Drench for oral administration (10%)

<u>Dose</u>: 7.5 mg/kg routine worming.
    30 mg/kg for cyathostomes.
    60 mg/kg for migrating strongyle larvae strongyles (or 7.5 mg/kg daily for 5 days, or 15 mg/kg daily for 4 days).
    15 mg/kg for D arnfieldi.
    prn

<u>Notes</u>: Resistance known to occur (monitor worm egg counts). Very safe.

Febantel: PML
  Bayverm [*Bayer*]

Indications: Broad spectrum anthelmintic. Possible effects on tapeworms?

Forms: Drench (2.5%) and pellets (1.9%) for oral administration

Dose: 6 mg/kg PO prn

Notes: Treatment of equine tapeworms with this has not been established.

Haloxon: PML
  Equilox# [*Crown*], Multiwurma* [*Day Son and Hewitt*]

Indications: Broad spectrum anthelmintic. Possible effects on tapeworms?

Forms: * Sachets containing 25 g. Tubs of 0.5/1 kg with 25 g
  # 10g in graduated (Kg) syringe for oral administration

Dose: * 50-70 mg/kg bodyweight mixed in feed
  # 22 mg/kg PO prn

Notes: Do not combine with other organophosphates. Do not use in first 4 weeks of pregnancy. 8 day withdrawal before racing.
NOT effective against equine tapeworms. Environmental considerations (Chickens/fish etc).

Ivermectin: PML
  Eqvalan [*MSD Agvet*]

Indications: Treatment / control of all major helminth parasites including lungworm. Treatment of hypobiotic larvae, lice and mange. Treatment of cutaneous and gastric Habronemiasis, Thelaziasis. Treatment and control of Bots.

Forms: Paste for oral administration in graduated syringe (kg) (1.87%w/w).

Dose: 200 μg/kg PO prn

Notes: Parenteral administration may cause severe life threatening reactions. IV use has been reported to be safe but not licensed. Injectable form may be given PO at 200μg/kg.
NOT effective against equine tapeworms. Environmental considerations.

Levamisole: PML
  Nemicide/Nilverm [*ICI*], Levacide [*Norbrook*]

Indications: Treatment / control of adult strongyles. Possible immune stimulatory properties
(intractable infections and immune compromise).

Forms: 7.5% solution for sc injection, oral drench (1.5% w/v)

Dose: Anthelmintic at 7.5 mg/kg PO prn.
  Immunostimulant 2mg/kg q 24h for 7 - 10 day repeated prn.

Notes: Anthelmintic effects poor (useful in treatment of lungworm in donkeys)

Mebendazole: PML
  Telmin [*Janssen*]

Indications: Treatment of helminthiasis (Strongyles and Cyathostomes), mature and larval
Parascaris equorum, adult Oxyuris equi, Dictyocaulus arnfieldi at special dose rate).

Forms: Graduated (kg) syringes containing 4g micronised mebendazole in 20 g paste.
  Sachets containing 2 g mebendazole for in feed use.

Dose: 5 - 10 mg/kg. Repeat every 6 weeks.
           15 - 20 mg/kg daily for 5 days for Dictyocaulus arnfieldi

Notes: Safe for pregnant mares and foals. May cause mild diarrhoea if overdosed.
Pregnant donkeys should NOT receive the higher dose regime.
Not for use in horses intended for human consumption. Resistance pattern not yet clear.

Metriphonate: PML
  Neguvon-P [*Bayer*]

Indications: Treatment of Gastrophilus sp (Bots), mature and larval Parascaris equorum, adult
Oxyuris equi.

Forms: Single dose graduated (kg) syringes (2.1 g) for oral dosing.

Dose: 35 mg/kg PO.

Notes: Administer 20 min before feeding. Do not exceed calculated dose. Ensure administration
onto top of tongue (not into pouches of cheeks or under tongue). May cause local reaction.
Pregnant mares and foals < 3 mths old should not be treated.
Rare side effects of trembling, sweating, colic, salivation etc. Do not treat with atropine unless
severe! Do not exercise for 48 hrs.
Environmental hazards to fish, birds and wildlife.

Oxfendazole: PML
   Synanthic [*Syntex*], Systamex [*Coopers*]

   Indications: Treatment / prophylaxis of ascarids, strongyles, Oxyuris equi, and adult T axei.

   Forms: Oral paste in graduated (kg) syringe (18.5% w/w),
        Pellets for in feed administration (6.8% w/v)

   Dose: 10 mg/kg PO prn

   Notes: Possible cross resistance with fenbendazole or specific resistance. Safe.

Oxibendazole: PML
   Equidin [*Univet*], Equitac [*Smith Kline*]

   Indications: Routine anthelmintic treatment and control.

   Forms: Oral paste in graduated (kg) syringes (8g as 30% w/w)

   Dose: 10 mg/kg PO prn

   Notes: Possible cross resistance or specific resistance with fenbendazole.

Piperazine BP: GSL

   Indications: Treatment of Parascaris equorum and adult strongyles (large and small).

   Forms: Powder for oral dosing
        Paste in graduated (Kg) syringe; oral

   Dose: 200 mg/kg (adipate /citrate) Maximum 30 g for foal, 80 g adults.

   Notes: No effect on migrating larvae.

Praziquantel: POM
   Droncit [*Bayer*]

   Indications: Tapeworm treatment

   Forms: 50 mg tablet oral

   Dose: 5 mg/kg

   Notes: Very expensive! Useful if Pyrantel ineffective.
        Not tested yet! Do not use injectable formulation.

Pyrantel embonate :   POM
Strongid [*Pfizer*]

Indications: Treatment/control of strongyles, oxyuris, parascaris. Also (at higher dose) effective against Paranoplocephala spp.

Forms: Oral paste in graduated syringe (kg) 10.36 g in 30 ml base
Powder/granules for in feed administration (76.7% w/w)

Dose: 19 mg /kg routine. 40 mg/kg for treatment of tapeworms.

Notes: Safe. No known resistance. Good efficacy against equine tapeworms.

Thiabendazole: PML
Equizole Pony Paste [*MSD Agvet*], Equizole Powder [*MSD Agvet*]

Indications: Treatment of adult helminth parasites. At higher doses effective against migrating strongyle larvae and lungworm.

Forms: Drench (suspension) for oral administration 17.6% w/v.
Paste for oral administration in graduated syringe (kg) 49.3%

Dose: Routine worming 44 mg/kg PO prn
Foal Ascariasis 88 mg/kg PO prn
Larvicidal (and lungworm) dose 440 mg/kg PO prn

Notes: Dose of 20 mg /kg PO q 24 h for 7 - 14 days has some antifungal properties.

b) Antibiotics:

Note: Every precaution should be taken to ensure responsible use of antibiotic compounds by the use of swabs, cultures and sensitivity testing of bacteria. Resistance in vitro does not always mean that the compound is of no value but due note must be taken of such results. Sensitivity in vivo, likewise may not result in sensitivity in vitro. Tissue availability of the compound may alter the effects significantly. Doses should be accurately calculated from the body weight of the patient and courses should be completed to avoid resistance as far as possible.
Commercial preparations containing more than one antibiotic agent may require dosage adjustment for one or other of the drugs included. It may be impossible to give the correct dosage of both or all the agents.

<u>Ampicillin</u>:   POM
Penbritin [*Beecham*], Duphacillin [*Duphar*], Compropen [*Pitman-Moore*], Embacillin[*RMB*], Amfipen [*Gistes-Brocades*], Norobrittin [*Norbrook*],

<u>Indications</u>: Infections due to Gram +ve organisms (except penicillinase producers) and most Gram -ve organisms (poor for E Coli)

<u>Presentation</u>: 500 mg powder for reconstitution single dose vials.
                        150 mg /ml suspension for IM injection 50/100 ml multidose vials

<u>Dose</u>: 10 - 50 mg /kg sodium salt (IV/IM) q 6 - 12 h
            5 - 10 mg/kg trihydrate salt (IM) q 12 - 24 h

<u>Notes</u>: Higher dose for serious infections, low for urinary tract infections.
Soluble salt only stable for 1-2 hours after reconstitution.
Bioavailablity high PO (Impractical po in all but foals).
Long acting contra-indicated (SEVERE LOCAL REACTIONS/ ANAPHYLAXIS)

<u>Chloramphenicol</u>:   POM
Salophen Co[*Arnolds*] (with dexamethasone and tripelenamine), Duphenicol [*Duphar*], Diochlor [*Millpledge*], Animycetin [*Intervet*],

<u>Indications</u>: Suspected/**confirmed** chloramphenicol sensitive Salmonellosis. Broad spectrum, bacteriostatic. CNS infections. Corneal ulceration (topical).

<u>Presentation</u>: 150/250 mg /ml solution for IV (IM) injection
                        Ophthalmic ointment (see ophthalmic drugs)

<u>Dose</u>: 25 - 50 mg/kg q 8/12 h IV (succinate preferred)

<u>Notes</u>: Rare aplastic anaemia in some humans. USE with extreme caution. Prolonged courses may result in reversible aplastic anaemia in horses. Significant interactions with penicillin and rifampicin.

Erythromycin:
   Erythromid [*Abbott*], Eryrthrocin Injectable [*CEVA Ltd*]

Indications: Macrolide -static or -cidal activity according to dose rate /susceptibility. Effective Gram +ve organisms, chlamydia, mycoplasma, listeria, rhodococcus, coryne

Presentation: Erythromycin estolate 250 mg caps, 500 mg tabs, 250 mg/5ml oral suspension. Water-miscible solution for injection 200 mg/ml in 50 ml multidose vial

Dose: 10 - 15 mg /kg PO q 8h.
* With Rifampicin -- use 15 mg/kg q 8h for up to 4 weeks or more.

Notes: Avoid if hepatic function not normal. Estolate best po.
AVOID PARENTERAL FORMS-- severe local reactions!

Gentamycin: POM
   Gentovet [*Arnolds*], Gentocin [*Schering*], Gentamicin inj BP [*Nicholas*],
   Pangram [*Virbac*]

   <u>Indications</u>: Infections due to most Gram +ve organisms. Particularly Ps aeruginosa, R equi.
   Bactericidal.

   <u>Presentation</u>: 20 / 40 mg /ml single dose (2ml) vials
               50 mg/ml multi dose (10ml/20ml/50ml) vials

   <u>Dose</u>: 3 mg/kg q 8 h IM (reactions!) or slow IV (10 mins)

   <u>Notes</u>: Good joint penetration. Nephrotoxic (prolonged courses). Foals < 4 mo may show severe
   nephrotoxicity. Monitor renal function before and during therapy. DO NOT USE WITH OTHER
   NEPHROTOXIC DRUGS. Risk of neuromuscular blockade.
   Poor oral absorbtion. Rapid resistance.

Kannamycin: POM

   <u>Indications</u>: Gram -ve bacterial infections.

   <u>Presentation</u>: 1 gr powder for reconstitution im injection

   <u>Dose</u>: 10 mg/kg IM q 12h

   <u>Notes</u>: Low risk nephrotoxicity

Neomycin: POM
   Penicillin-Neomycin [*Intervet*](with procaine penicillin), Neobiotic [*Upjohn*]

   <u>Indications</u>: Gram -ve infections (especially enteric organisms)
   Ophthalmic infections

   <u>Presentation</u>: Solution for injection 50/100/200 mg/ml 100 ml multidose vials
   Ophthalmic cream (see ophthalmic drugs below)

   <u>Dose</u>: 5 - 10 mg /kg IM q 12 - 24h

   <u>Notes</u>: Toxic effects as for gentamycin.
   Useful for R equi infection if rifampicin resistance. May be given PO in foals (check suitable
   formulation).

Nitrofurantoin:
Berkfurin-E [*Berk*]

Indications: Broad spectrum bactericidal effect. Urinary and respiratory tract bacterial infections.

Presentation: Pale yellow powder (50% w/w) in palatable base for oral administration, single dose sachets (1 gr each)

Dose: 20 mg/kg (2 sachets initially for 450 kg horse), one sachet PO q 8 h 5 - 7 days

Notes: Occasional urticarial skin reactions (stop course)

Penicillin (Benzathine, G-K, G-Na, G-procaine):
Depopen [*Gistes-Brocade*], Depocillin [*Gistes-Brocade*],
Duplocillin [*Gistes-Brocade*], Mylipen [*Pitman-Moore*], Propen [*Pitman-Moore*],
Crystapen [*Pitman-Moore*], Streptopen (with streptomycin) [*Pitman-Moore*],
Streptovin (with streptomycin and betamethasone) [*Pitman-Moore*], Diopen [*Alan Hitchins*],
Procillin[*Bimeda*], Ilcocillin [*Ciba-Geigy*], Vetipen [*C-Vet*], Duphapen [*Duphar*],
Ethacillin [*Intervet*], Milimycin (with streptomycin)[*Intervet*],
Lenticillin [*RMB*], Lentrax [*RMB*], Depopen [*BK Prod*],
Depomycin (with streptomycin)[*BK Prod*], Norocillin [*Norbrook*],
Norocillin LA [*[Norbrook*], Vidopen[*BK Prod*], etc.

Indications: Infections due to penicillin sensitive Gram +ve bacteria.

Presentation:

FORM	routes	forms*	dose
Na benzyl pen	IM (IV#)	1/5g vials	10-20 mg/kg (1000 - 1500 iu/kg) q8h
Procaine pen	IM	100 ml m-d 300mg/ml	10-25 mg/kg (1500 - 2000 iu/kg) q24h
Benzathine pen	IM	100 ml m-d 150mg/ml	15-30 mg/kg (1500 - 2000 iu/kg) q48h

*Note many formulations are in iu/ml.

Dose: see above

Notes: #IV Na^+ or K^+ benzathine penicillin occasionally associated with sudden death and /or cardiac arrhythmias. Do not give during anaesthesia or in combination with other drugs likely affecting cardiac rhythm. Na^+ salts absorbed more slowly when given IM. Avoid concurrent use of bacteriostatic antibiotics. Do not mix with other drugs in syringe.
Allergies possible (anaphylactic reactions - if these are encountered do not use cephalosporins either). Treat with adrenaline etc.

Warning: Check contents/permitted route before use (many products are cocktails of drugs!). Mixtures of different drugs may make accurate dosage of all components difficult!

Rifampicin: POM
  Rifampin [*Abbott*], Rifadin/Rifadin for Infusion [*Merrell Dow*], Rimactane [*Ciba*]

  Indications: Broad spectrum antibiotic. Particularly indicated for Rhodococcus equi (with erythromycin). Treatment of TB.

  Presentation: 300 mg capsule, Oral
              20 ml vial single dose (600mg) for infusion

  Dose: 10 mg/kg PO q 12h. Infusion given at 20 mg/kg over 3-4 hours.

  Notes: Rapid resistance; use with erythromycin (qv) (synergistic effect). Excellent lipid solubility and cell/tissue penetrating properties.
  May cause red discoloration in urine. Very safe even over long courses.
  Expensive.

Streptomycin: POM
  Dimicin [*Pitman-Moore*], Streptopen [*Pitman-Moore*](with procaine penicillin),
  Streptovin [*Pitman-Moore*](with procaine penicillin and dexamethasone),
  Penstrep [*C-Vet*](with procaine penicillin),

  Indications: Streptomycin sensitive bacterial infections (Gram -ve mostly), Staphylococcal infections.

  Presentation: Solution for im 250 mg/ml injection

  Dose: 10 mg/kg IM (IV) q 12h

  Notes: Slight risk nephrotoxicity/oto-toxicity

c) Sulphonamides:

Sulphadimidine:
Sulphamezathine [*Rhone Merieux*], Sulphadimidine [*Peter Hand*]

Indications: Treatment of bacterial infections of upper respiratory tract

Presentation: Free flowing white crystalline powder for oral administration

Dose: 100 mg/kg PO in feed q 12 h 5 - 7 days

Notes: Ensure good water intake. Prolonged courses use 50 mg/kg and administer B complex vitamins parenterally

Trimethoprim Sulphonamides: POM
Tribrissen[*Coopers*], Trivetrin [*Coopers*], Duphatrim [*Duphar*],
Borgal [*Hoechst*], Equitrim [*Boehringer Ingelheim*]

Indications: Broad spectrum antibacterial (most gram -ve and some Gram +ve). Protozoal encephalomyelitis.

Presentation: 24% / 48% solution for IM or IV injection 50/100 ml multidose vials. 48% suspension for im injection 100 ml multidose vials.
30 gram syringe for oral dosing (graduated /kg)
Single dose sachets (12gr) (one /500 kg) oral

Dose: 24 mg (combined active ingredients)/kg IV/IM/PO q 12 h
(equivalent to **4 and 20 mg/kg trimethoprim/sulphadoxine** respectively)

Notes: Ps. aeruginosa resistant. Oral courses effective over long periods without apparent toxic effects. Check formulation and permitted route before adminstration.

114

d) Other Antibacterials:

Metronidazole: POM
Torgyl Forte [*Rhone Merieux*], Torgyl Solution [*Rhone Merieux*]
Flagyl Tbs [*Rhone Merieux*]

Indications: Anaerobic systemic and local infections, protozoal infections. Good oral absorbtion and tissue penetration.

Forms: 500 mg tablet, oral
    5 mg /ml sterile solution IV (50ml single dose plastic sachets)

Dose: Torgyl Solution 20 - 40 mg/kg IV q 8 -12 h (NOT SC)
    Torgyl Forte 20- 40 mg/kg IM ONLY

Notes: Solutions not specifically prepared for IV injection should be filtered as administered by slow IV injection. Read data sheet before administration!
Soaked swabs may control local anaerobic infections eg feet/wounds.

e) Antifungal agents

Amphoteracin B:

Indications: Deep or systemic mycoses. Histoplasmosis, Blastomycosis

Presentation: 50 mg/ml injection single dose vials

Dose: 10 mg test dose. 0.2 mg/kg increasing to 0.5 - 1.0 mg/kg over 2 days. Given as very dilute IV solution (0.1 mg/ml in 5% dextrose saline drip)

Notes: Very light sensitive (protected from light at all times).
Nephrotoxicity common if prolonged course. May be given alternate days to reduce toxic effects. Monitor renal function. Dilute to avoid cardiac toxicity.
May be given with corticosteroids to reduce adverse effects during administration.

Benzuldasic Acid:
Defungit [*Hoechst*]

Indications: External treatment of dermatomycoses.

Forms: White amorphous powder, non irritant external wash. 10 gr sachets

Dose: 0.5% solution applied externally (1 sachet in 2 l water) prn q 48 h

Notes: Also has some bacteriostatic properties. No need to remove scales and crusts. Use as wash applied with sponge or spray. Use solution promptly.

Griseofulvin:
Fulcin [*Coopers*], Grisovin [*Pitman-Moore*],
Equifulvin Paste and Granules[*Boehringer Ingelheim*]

Indications: Systemic treatment of dermatomycoses

Forms: Fine beige powder containing 7.5% griseofulvin. 1 kg and 3.5 kg packs with 20g and 100 g dispensing cups included. Paste in graduated dosing syringe for oral use (33%)

Dose: 130 mg/kg (10 g /75 kg) PO q 24 h for 10 - 14 days

Notes: Not to be used during pregnancy. Reduced effect if intercurrent PBZ.
Effect slow to develop.
No action against systemic mycoses due to Candida, Aspergillus, blastomycoses, etc.
Should not be handled by women of child bearing age.

Miconazole: POM
Imaverol [*Janssen*], Conoderm [*C Vet*]

Indications: Topical treatment of dermatomycoses

Forms: Oily liquid 100 mg/ml concentrate, 100ml and 1l bottles
Cream 23 mg/g for topical application.

Dose: Prepared as 0.2% emulsion(1:50), apply to lesions and immediate surrounds 3-4 times daily at 3 day intervals. Topical cream applied to lesions once daily for up to 6 weeks.

Notes: Remove crusts before use.

Natamycin: POM
Mycophyte [*Mycofarm*]

Indications: Topical and environmental treatment of dermatomycoses

Forms: Dry powder for re-suspension containing 1 g /10 g powder. Bottles containing 2 and 10 g

Dose: 10 l water (10g bottle) to suspend carefully. Sponge onto skin or spray. Wood, leather and metal can be sprayed. Repeat after 4 - 5 days.

Notes: Very safe.

f) Antiprotozoal:

POM

Diminazene Aceturate:
  Berenil [*Hoechst*]

Indications: Treatment of babesiosis due to B equi and B caballi. Treatment of trypanosomiasis (including Dourine [T equiperdum] and Surra [T brucei]).

Forms: Powder (1.05g) in sachets for reconstitution (12.5 ml water) as non sterile 7% solution for injection.

Dose: 3.5 mg/kg deep im single dose only.
  7.0 mg/kg for treatment of Trypanosoma brucei infection.

Notes: Severe local reactions including abscessation, sloughing etc are common. Anaphylactic reactions have resulted in peracute death. Very low therapeutic index.

POM

Imidocarb:
  Imazole [*Pitman-More*]

Indications: Treatment of babesiosis due to B equi and B caballi.

Forms: 12% solution for injection 50 ml multidose vials

Dose: 2mg/kg deep im q 24h on two consecutive days

Notes: Severe local reactions are common.

Metronidazole: see Antibacterials (p114)

g) Parasiticides

Coumaphos: (PML)
Asuntol Louse Powder [*Bayer*]

Indications: Ectoparasiticide for control of lice

Forms: 1% powder in Shaker

Dose: Repeat at 14 day interval (NOT LESS)

Notes: For topical treatment only. Care with handling should be taken.

Cypermethrin: (PML)
Rycopel [*Rycovet Ltd*]

Indications: Ectoparasiticide for control of nuisance flies such as H irritans, H bovis, G intestinalis etc

Forms: 5% emulsifiable concentrate

Dose: Diluted 1: 50 with water used as TOPICAL WASH. Applied to mane neck etc at sites of predilection for flies. Repeated 14-28 days.

Notes: For topical treatment only. Care with handling should be taken.

Gamma Benzene Hexachloride (BHC): PML
ICI Louse and Insect powder [*Pitman More/ICI*], Lorexane [*Pitman More/ICI*]

Indications: Ectoparasite control. Lice, mites, ticks

Forms: Powder for suspension as wash for topical application.

Dose: Wash repeated pnr

Notes: Safe but environmentally less desirable.

Lindane: (GSL)

Sweet Itch Solution [*Day Son and Hewitt*]

Indications: Ectoparasiticide for control of Sweet Itch

Forms: 0.1% solution

Dose: as required. Human toxic effects (WEAR GLOVES etc)

Monosulfiram: (PML)

Tetmosol [*ICI*]

Indications: Ectoparasiticide with some antifungal properties

Forms: Soap block

Dose: prn

Notes: Non toxic and non irritant.

NOTES

NOTES

NOTES

SECTION 8: *BLOOD MODIFYING AGENTS:*

a) Anticoagulants:

Calcium Gluconate: N/C

Indications: Control of intravascular thrombosis

Presentation: Dry powder

Dose: 500 - 600 mg/kg as 20% solution by very slow IV

Notes: Usually use 1.5 l of 20% solution IV. Results equivocal in treatment of aorto-iliac thrombosis. (ref: Branscome, 1968: JAVMA 152 1643)
May be antagonised with VITAMIN K₁

Heparin Sodium: POM
Heparin [*Boots*], Heparin Injection BP [*CP Pharm's*]

Indications: Prevents formation of stable fibrin clots.
Thromboembolism, Disseminated Intravascular Coagulopathy (DIC), prevention of *in vitro* or *in vivo* coagulation. Prevention of abdominal adhesions following laparotomy.

Presentation: Heparin Na 1,000, 5000, 10,000, 25,000 iu/ml as 1 - 5 ml multidose vials.

Dose: Anticoagulation: 25 - 100 iu/kg q 4 h IV
Peritoneal lavage: 50 iu/kg in lavage solution
Catheter management: 1,000 iu in 100ml (10iu/ml)

Notes: Combines with **Antithrombin iii** to inactivate **Factor Xa** and prevent conversion of prothrombin. At high doses inactivates **thrombin** - inhibits **Factors IX, X, XI, XII, XIII**. No effect on clotting factor concentrations. **Does not lyse clots!**
IV only! IM may cause haematomas. May be given by constant IV infusion.
Specific antagonist PROTAMINE SULPHATE.

Protamine Sulphate: POM

Indications: Anticoagulant when given alone. When given with heparin stable salt is formed (reducing anticoagulant effects of both). Antagonises effect of heparin Sulphate within 5 min. Effect duration approx. 2 hours.

Presentation: 10 mg/ml injection (25 ml multidose vial)

Dose: 1 mg Protamine inactivates 100 iu heparin sulphate. Max dose 100 mg very slowly IV.

Notes: Beware of anaphylaxis. Incompatible with benzyl and procaine penicillins

Warfarin: POM
    Marevan [*Duncan, Flockart & Co*]

    Indications: Thrombotic conditions including NAVICULAR DISEASE

    Presentation: 1 mg, 3 mg, 5 mg tablets ORAL

    Dose: 0.05 - 0.1 mg /kg PO q 24 h

    Notes: Gradual onset of effect.
Test FIRST STAGE PROTHROMBIN TIME before instigating programme and monitor regularly. Treatment for ND: maintain steady 50% increase in PT. Variations may occur related to dietary intake, work and other medications.
Do not use with phenylbutazone or other non-steroidals likely to induce ulceration of stomach or intestinal tract.

b) Coagulants

Malonic/Oxalic Acid: POM
  Venagmin [*Willows Francis*]

  Indications: Epistaxis, uterine/enteric bleeding, Purpura haemorrhagica

  Presentation: Aqueous solution containing 2.5 mg Malonic Acid and 7.5 mg Oxalic Acid /ml.
  30ml multidose vial.

  Dose: 10-20 ml IV / IM

  Notes: Poorly defined effects. Equivocal efficacy.

Menadione: POM
  Vitamin K_3

  Indications: Anaemia

  Presentation: Injection 50 mg/ml Menadione Na Bisulphite (multidose vials)

  Dose: 2 - 4 mg /kg IM/SC

  Notes: May induce tubular nephrosis ---- use low doses
  Slow onset of effects. For immediate effects in antagonising warfarin (qv) use Vit K_1
  (Phytomenadione)(qv).

Phytomenadione/Vitamin K1:   POM
  Konakion [*Roche*]

  Indications: Antagonist for warfarin overdose, haemorrhage, anaemia

  Presentation: 10 mg/ml ampoules (1ml)

  Dose: 75 mg q 12 h SC/IM/IV

c) Haematinics:

Most haematinics are compounds of Vitamins and Minerals (see Vitamin Preparations)

d) Vitamin preparations:

Vitamin B1 (Thiamine HCl):
Vitamin B_1 Injection [*Bimeda*], Parentrovite (with other B vits) [*Beecham*]

Indications: Bracken poisoning, Exertional rhabdomyolysis

Presentation: 100 mg/ml aqueous solution 50 ml multidose vial

Dose: 10mg /kg slow IV or IM injection q 4hr

Notes: IV injections may result in anaphylactic reactions. Avoid if possible - use very slow IV.

Vitamin B12:
Vit B_{12} Forte Inj, Vitbee 1000, DiovitB12, Intravit 12,
Vitamin B_{12} Injection 1000mcg/ml,

Indications: Vitamin B_{12} deficiency conditions, anaemia

Presentation: 1000 μg/ml aqueous solution, 5, 20 50 ml multidose vials

Dose: 1000 - 5000 μg total dose IM, weekly prn

Notes: May also have metabolic stimulant properties

Biotin:

Kerafac []

Indications: Foot care supplement

Forms: Oral powder

Dose:

Notes: Often mixed with other vitamin/mineral supplementations

Methionine BP:

Indications: Treatment of refractory laminitis and poor hoof quality. Hoof wall defects. Re-establishment of depleted keratin sulphate.

Forms: 99% powder or in feed palatable cubettes.

Dose: 22 mg/kg po in feed q 24h for 1 - 3 weeks, may be halved for subsequent weeks after first. (10 g daily for 1 week, 5 g daily for 3-4 weeks)

Notes: Safe but unreliable/poorly documented benefit

Vitamin B Complex:

Parentrovite(with Ascorbic Acid BP) [*Beecham*],

Haemo-15 (with Iron, Vit B12, Copper, Cobalt, biotin, innositol, methionine, lysine) [*Arnolds*]

Indications: Stress, toxic or deficiency conditions. Supportive therapy.

Forms: Aqueous solution of Thiamine BP, Riboflavine BP, Pyridoxine BP, nicotinamide BP, minerals and amino acids for injection

Dose: Various doses according to concentrations 10 - 20 - 30 ml IV (very slowly) or IM, q 24 h, repeat 3 days

Notes: Preparations containing Thiamine may cause anaphylactic shock in some animals. Slow IV (should be diluted with saline). Do not mix with other substances. IM injection may result in large local reactions. Haemo-15 does not contain Thiamine.
CHECK contents of formulation/product before using!

Vitamin E / Selenium:

Dystosel [*Intervet*], Selenavite E and other dietary supplements.
Indications: Prophylaxis and treatment of Selenium and Vitamin E deficiency syndromes including nutritional muscular dystrophy, recurrent Tying Up syndrome etc.

Forms: White sterile suspension containing 1.5 mg K selenate and 68 iu Vit E /ml for im use. Various forms for oral use.

Dose: 5 ml total dose for 500 kg horse. Repeat weekly.

Notes: Dubious benefit! Monitor blood levels before and during treatment. May cause marked local reaction.

e) Electrolytes/Fluids:

Parenteral Fluids Comparison Table: (milliequivalents/litre)

Solution	Na	K	Ca	Mg	Cl	Lact	HCO3
Normal saline	154				154		
Ringers	147	4	4.5		156		
Ringer/Lactate (Hartmans)	130	4	3		109	28	
5% Na Bicarbonate	595						595

To make:
1 litre Normal saline : 9g NaCl in 1000ml water (pyrogen free)

1 litre Hartmans:

	Na Lactate	3.1 g
	Na Chloride	6.0 g
	K Chloride	0.3 g
	Ca Chloride.2H₂O	0.2 g
	Water	qs 1000ml

1 litre Molar Bicarbonate: 85 gr NaHCO₃ per litre water

1 litre Isotonic Bicarbonate: 12.5 g NaHCO₃ per litre water

1 litre Isotonic Dextrose: 50g dextrose (or 100ml 50% solution) per litre water

1 litre Ca gluconate : 200 g Ca gluconate
                40 g Boric Acid   Water qs 1000ml

1 litre Isotonic Potassium Chloride (146 meq/l): 11 g K Chloride per litre water

1 litre 7% (hypertonic) Saline 7 g NaCl + water qs 1000ml

Heparin-Saline: 2500 iu Heparin Na in 500 ml saline (Discard after 1 week max)

NOTES: Self-prepared electrolytes must be sterile and prepared with pyrogen free distilled or deionised water.

Total Blood Volume = 80 - 90 mls/ kg

Metabolic Fluid Requirement = 15 ml / kg / day

Fluid Deficit (mls) = 10x % dehydration x body weight

Bicarbonate Deficit (mmol OR mls 8.4%) = 0.3 x Base excess x Body Weight (kg)
Note: Bicarbonate should only be administered when Base Excess is negative, pH is acidic and plasma bicarbonate is low - ie in metabolic acidosis. Bicarbonate is contraindicated in respiratory acidosis.
Note: Suitable Analytical Reagent chemicals (AnalaR) from BDH/MERCK/SIGMA/ALDRICH

Colloidal IV Solutions:
    Haemaccel [*Hoechst*], Onkovertin [*B.Braun*]

    Indications: Life-threatening circulatory shock. For rapid blood volume replacement therapy, especially when total protein is low < 30 g/dl.

    Presentation: 500ml plastic containers

    Dose: Usually used with crystalloids. Administer until desired improvement in cardiovascular function is seen.
    Up to 10mls/kg/hour can be safely administered. Total daily dose 40mls/kg

    Notes: Retained in circulation for 2- 3 hours. Renal excretion occurs.
    Contraindicated in acute renal failure.

Gelatins:
    Gelofusin Vet. [*Consolidated Chemicals Ltd*]

    Presentation: As above

    Dose: As above

    Notes: As above. Considerably less expensive than Haemaccel and equally as efficacious.

Dextrans: Dextran 70 *(Macrodex, Pharmacia)*.

    Presentation: Macrodex 6% in dextrose and Macrodex 6% in saline. 500mls single use bottles.

    Dose: Not > 5mls/kg/hr, to avoid thrombasthenic haemorrhagic diathesis. Total daily dose 40 mls/kg

    Notes: As above. Increases plasma volume by 60 - 70 % above infused volume (cf 50% other colloids). Refractometric index of 46 g/l. Half life 12 - 24 hours.
    If bleeding occurs, cease administration.
    Large infusions interfere with red cell antigen cross-matching.

Starches:
    Hydoxyethyl Starch *(Hetastarch)*

    Indications: As Above

    Dose: As above. Do not exceed 30mls/kg/day

    Notes: Can cause bleeding. Interferes with antigen/antibody testing. Lasts 24-36h Very expensive.

Parenteral feeding Fluids:

Duphalyte [*Duphar*].

Indications: Injectable solution of electrolytes, vitamins, amino acids and dextrose, Support therapy in animals.

Forms: Plastic bottles of yellow solution 500mls

Dose: up to 100mls per 50kg bodyweight q 24 - 48h

Notes: **Slow** iv only. Not sufficient for daily fluid maintenance requirements or for total intravenous nutrition. **Supportive treatment only.**

NOTES

SECTION 9: *VACCINES / ANTISERA*

NOTES

African Horse Sickness Vaccine:

Indications: Prophylaxis for African Horse Sickness

Forms: Freeze dried pellet of live virus particles of modified strains (8 Strains included covers 43 antigenic types). Reconstituted with water provided. Single dose vials 5 ml.

Dose: 5ml IM VACCINE 1, followed 4 weeks later by 5 ml IM VACCINE 2. Annual boosters may be as above but may be combined as single dose.

Notes: Poor efficacy, REST imperative for entire course. Some severe reactions.

EHV, Vaccine:
Pneumobort K [ScanVet UK]

Indications: Prevention of EHV, abortion in healthy mares and in contact horses

Forms: Formaldehyde inactivated virus in oily adjuvant, single dose pre-filled syringes

Dose: 2ml IM in 5th, 7th and 9th month of pregnancy. Non -pregnant animals of all sexes should receive 2 doses at 4-6 week intervals with boosters every 6 months.

Notes: Severe local reactions follow accidental self-injection. EMERGENCY MEDICAL HELP MUST BE SOUGHT IMMEDIATELY! (inform doctor that oily vaccine)

Influenza Vaccine:
  Prevac [*Hoechst*], Prevac T (with Tetanus Toxoid) [*Hoechst*],
  Duvaxyn [*Duphar*], Duvaxyn IE-T [*Duphar*](with Tetanus Toxoid),
  Eqinplus-T [*Coopers*], Eqinplus-T [*Coopers*](with Tetanus Toxoid),

Indications: Prophylactic vaccination for Equine Influenza

Forms: 2 ml single dose vials for injection

Name	Prague (IA/E1)	Kentucky (IA/E2)	Miami (IA/E2)	Fontainbleau (IA/E2)
Prevac/T	*		*	*
Duvaxyn/IE-t	*	*	*	
Equinplus/t	*	*	*	

Dose: Single dose 1 ml vials or preloaded syringes IM

Notes: JOCKEY CLUB (FIE / BHS) REGULATIONS:
  First Primary   Day 0
  Second Primary   21 - 90 days after first
  Booster Primary   150 - 190 days from second
  Annual Booster   ≤ 365 days

If overdue (even by 1 day) whole course to start again. Anniversary acceptable. No horse may be presented at a race meeting whose vaccination was given less than 10 days previously.

Foals : start around 4 - 6 months
BOOSTERS : recommended at 6 - 9 months intervals

NOTE: Horses rested for 2 - 4 days before and 4 - 10 days after vaccination (if not risk of myocarditis, pps etc).
Some reports of persistent coughing/Poor Performance Syndrome after vaccination.
Do not contaminate needles/syringes. Do not mix with other products.
Occasional anaphylaxis (treat with adrenaline)
DOES NOT PREVENT ALL RESPIRATORY DISEASE!
Most outbreaks due to IA/E2 strains. Note antigenic drift.

Tetanus Antiserum: POM

Equitoxin [*Coopers*], Tetanus Toxoid (BvetC)[*Coopers*], Tetanus Antitoxin [*Pitman More*]
Tetanus Antitoxin [*Hoechst*], Tetanus Antitoxin [*C-Vet*]

Indications: Prophylaxis and treatment of tetanus.

Forms: Refined concentrated hyperimmune serum produced in horses containing 500 - 3,000
iu.ml in prefilled syringes or 50 ml multidose vials.

Dose: Prophylaxis: 3,000 - 6,000 iu (total) SC or slow IV single dose lasts 4 -5 weeks
   Treatment: 100,000 - 250,000 iu IV +/- intrathecal injection, repeated daily prn

Notes: Anaphylaxis possible (rare). Care with asepsis. Effective cover for 6 weeks.
   Do not use preopened bottles for intra-thecal use.

Tetanus Toxoid: POM

Thorovax [*Coopers*], Tetanus Toxoid [*Coopers*], Tetanus Toxoid [*C-Vet*]
PrevacT [*Hoechst*] (with equine influenza antigen),
Equinplus -T [*Coopers*] (with equine influenza antigen), Tetanus Toxoid [*Hoechst*]
Duvaxyn IE-T [*Duphar*](with equine influenza antigen),
Tetanus Toxoid Vet. [*Pitman-More*], Thorovax Tetanus Toxoid Equidae[*Pitman-More*]

Indications: Prophylaxis for tetanus

Forms: Single dose vials or preloaded syringes 1 ml injection

Dose: 1 ml dose given deep IM. Initial course : two doses 4 - 6 weeks apart. Booster given at 6
months then bi-annually.
Foals may be vaccinated from 6 weeks of age according to expected passive immune status.

Notes: Very safe/effective

NOTES

SECTION 10: *MISCELLANEOUS DRUGS*:

Including:

a) Local Anaesthetics

b) Eye Preparations

c) Skin Preparations

d) Joint Preparations

e) Antidotes

f) Suture Materials

NOTES

a) Local Anaesthetics:

Bupivicaine: POM
   Marcaine [*Astra*]

   Indications: Local, perineurial and regional anaesthesia.

   Forms: 0.5% solution in single use ampoules.

   Dose : As for 2% lignocaine

   Notes: Long duration of action up to 6 hours. Slightly slower onset of action.

Lignocaine HCl: POM
   Locovetic [*Bimeda UK*], Xylotox [*Willows Francis*], Lignavet [*C-Vet Ltd*],
   Lignavet Epidural [*C-Vet Ltd*], Lignavet Plus [*C-Vet Ltd*], Wilcain [*Dales Pharmaceuticals*]
   Locaine 2% [*Animalcare*], Lignol [*Arnolds*], Diocaine [*Alan Hitchins*],
   Lignocaine Injection [*Norbrook, Pharmavet, Univet*],

   Indications: Local analgesia, perineurial regional anaesthesia, epidural anaesthesia, IVRA, control
   of intra-operative cardiac fibrillation

   Forms: Aqueous 2% solution for injection. Sterile multidose vials.

   Dose: Variable according to site and purpose (see Nerve Block Sites: Page 133).
   Epidural anaesthesia use only 4 - 7 ml (small space).

   Notes: Check if **adrenaline** added to preparation. Use only specified forms for epidural use.
   Lasts 30 - 40 mins (2x with adrenaline added). Poor penetration through fascial planes so
   accurate placement important. Very stable solution (can be boiled without effect (nb adrenaline
   labile)

Mepivicaine: POM
   Intra-Epicaine [*Arnolds*], Carbocaine [*Pharmacia*]

   Indications: Amide local anaesthetic. Prolonged action. Little irritant/toxic effect in joints or
   epidural.

   Forms: 2% solution in sterile multidose (10, 20, 50ml) vials.

   Dose: Epidural: 3 - 5 ml (20 - 30 min onset)
      Regional: 3 - 20 ml (30 min onset)
      Intra-articular: 3 - 30 ml (15 min onset)

   Notes: Safe. Avoid IV. Duration approx 2 hours.

b) Eye Preparations:

i) antibiotics

Acyclovir/Isoxuridine: POM
Zovirax Ophthalmic Ointment [*Wellcome Medical*]

Profile: Treatment of viral (herpes) keratitis. White sterile ointment (3%) in 4.5g tube. Apply 1-2 cm ribbon q 4h. Transient mild discomfort.

Chloramphenicol: POM
Chloramphenicol Ophthalmic Ointment 1% [*Parke, Davis*], Chloromycetin- Hydrocortisone Ophthalmic Ointment (with 0.5% hydrocortisone)[*Parke, Davis*]
Minims Chloramphenicol / Sno*Phenicol (0.5%)[*Smith&Nephew*]

Profile: Potent broad spectrum (-cidal) antibiotic. White ointment (4 g tubes).
Use only for chloromycetin sensitive infections. Apply q 6 h(min) and continue until 48 hours after recovery.
USE GLOVES– risk of aplastic anaemia!
Preparations with hydrocortisone are contra-indicated in infective and

Gentamycin: POM
Minims Gentamycin SO₄ [*Smith&Nephew*]

Profile: Single use, 0.5 ml clear drops (0.3%). Broad spectrum antibiotic (including action against Pseudomonas spp). Apply 10-15 drops q 6 h pnr.

Neomycin: POM
Vetsovate Eye Drops/Betsolan Eye Drops (with betamethasone) [*Pitman More*]

Profile: Broad spectrum antibiotic used to provide antibiotic cover for betamethasone.
Use for treatment and control of bacterial infections of the eye. Apply 2-4 drops q 8h.
Preparations containing corticosteroids contra-indicated if infection/ulcers.

ii) midriatics

Atropine Sulphate BP: POM
Minims Atropine Sulphate [*Smith&Nephew*], Alcon Opulets*Atropine [*Alcon Labs*]

Profile: Drops (1%, 5%), Ointment 1%, 5%).
Prolonged mydriasis (5 - 7 days) may follow single dose. Indicated in treatment of Uveitis (P-O)
and other painful conditions of the eye. Keep patient out of direct sunlight (preferably in
darkened box). Consider Homatropine Bromide as mydriasis can be reversed with physostigmine.

Homatropine Bromide: POM
Minims Homatropine Bromide [*Smith&Nephew*]

Profile: Clear 2% solution as drops. 2-4 drops q6h. Mydriasis more rapid than atropine and
reversed with physostigmine. Keep patient out of direct sunlight (preferably in darkened box).

Phenylephrine: POM
Phenylephrine Drops [*Richard Daniels*], Minims Phenylephrine HCl [*Smith&Nephew*]

Profile: 2.5%, 10% aqueous solution for ophthalmic use. Marked but short acting mydriatic.
Indicated for uveitis / pain / glaucoma etc. Apply 2-4 drops q 4-6h. Keep patient out of direct
sunlight (preferably in darkened box). Rebound miosis/irritation/corneal oedema.

Tropicamide: POM
Minims Tropicamide [*Smith&Nephew*], Mydriacyl [*Alcon Labs*]

Profile: Clear 0.5%, 1% solution as drops. 2 - 5 drops q 1h pnr.

iii) <u>miotics</u>

<u>Physostigmine Salicylate BVetC</u>:   POM

<u>Profile</u>: 0.125% eye ointment, paper strip containing 0.06 mg
Applied q 12h pnr.
Useful in convalescent stages of periodic ophthalmia.

<u>Pilocarpine Nitrate</u>:   POM
Minims Pilocarpine Nitrate / Sno*Pilo [*Smith&Nephew*]
Isopto*carpine [*Alcon Labs*]

<u>Profile</u>: 1%, 2%, 4%, solution as drops. Potent miotic for reversing effects of midriatics. Apply
1 -2 drops q 5min until effect. effect may last >2 hr. Treatment of glaucoma.

iv) <u>topical anaesthetics</u>

<u>Amethocaine</u>:   POM
Amethazole (with sulphathiazole) [*J.M.Loveridge*],
Minims Amethocaine HCl [*Smith&Nephew*]

<u>Profile</u>: Free flowing ointment base 0.5% or 0.5%, 1% drops. Apply 1 - 5 drops pnr. Initial
discomfort. Protect eye from dust and trauma. Effect lasts 5 - 10 min.

<u>Oxybuprocaine HCl</u>:   POM
Minims Benoxinate HCl [*Smith&Nephew*], Alcon Opulets*Benoxinate [*Alcon Labs*]

<u>Profile</u>: 0.4% clear solution as drops. Apply 2 -6 drops. Fast acting (<1min but short (5min).
Prolonged use may result in ulceration.

<u>Proxymetacaine HCl</u>:   POM
(Opthaine [*E.R.Squibb & Sons*])

<u>Profile</u>: 0.5% solution for surface analgesia of the eye. Rapid onset (10secs) lasts for 15 mins)

v) Steroids

Betamethasone: POM
  Vetsovate Eye Drops/Betsolan Eye Drops (with betamethasone) [*Pitman More*]

  Profile: Anti-inflammatory with antibiotic to control infection.
  Use for treatment and control of corneal/conjunctival inflammation. Apply 2-4 drops q 8h.
  Preparations containing corticosteroids contra-indicated if infection/ulcers.
  CONTRAINDICATED in corneal ulceration/infective conditions

Dexamethasone: POM
  Maxidex [*Alcon Labs*], Maxitrol (with PolymixinB, Neomycin sulph)

  Profile: Sterile (0.5%) solution as drops (with Hypromellose). Steroid responsive conditions
  without ulceration or infection. Apply 2 - 4 drops q 4h pnr. Fungal or bacterial; overgrowth
  may be serious complication.

Hydrocortisone: POM
  Chloromycetin-Hydrocortisone Ointment (with 1% chloramphenicol)[*Parke, Davis*]

  Profile: Potent anti-inflammatory topical ointment. Used where reduction of inflammatory
  response is indicated in absence of ulceration.
  CONTRAINDICATED in corneal ulceration conditions

Phenylbutazone: POM
  Tanderil [*Zyma (UK) Ltd*], Tanderil with 1% Chloramphenicol [*Zyma(UK)*]

  Profile: Free flowing ointment for topical application containing 10 % oxyphenbutazone. Good
  penetration to anterior chamber and uveal tract. Useful as non steroidal anti-inflammatory. Useful
  as non steroidal! Uveitis treatment.
  Apply q 4-5h, pnr

vi) <u>Artificial Tears</u>:

<u>Hypromellose USP</u>:   POM
   Tears Naturelle [*Acon Labs*], Sno*Tears [*Smith&Nephew*]

<u>Profile</u>: 15 ml droppers containing hypromellose (0.3%) and dextran70. Used to provide
lubrication for eye where xerophthalmia or keratoconjunctivitis sicca present. Apply frequently (q
2-3h minimum) pnr.

*Note: Sterile saline may be effectively used to provide irrigation and lubrication. Water should
not be used.*

vii) <u>Ophthalmic Diagnostics & Miscellaneous Drugs</u>

<u>EDTA</u>:   not classified

> <u>Profile</u>: Anti-collagenase. Control and treatment of melting ulcers. Add 3 ml sterile saline to 10 ml <u>EDTA</u> Vacutainer (B-D Ltd)(ideally 2% solution of EDTA). Apply as drops q 2h.
> ALTERNATIVES: Solution of acetylcysteine or saliva.

<u>Fluorescein</u>:
> Minims Fluorescein Na / Minims Lignocaine + Fluorescein [*Smith&Nephew*]
> Alcon Opulets*Fluorescein Na [*Alcon Labs*], Fluorets [*Smith&Nephew*]

> <u>Profile</u>: Single use sterile drops (1%,2%) or impregnated paper strips (1mg). Diagnostic solution for detection of corneal ulceration and patency of naso-lacrimal duct (may take 5 - 15 min to pass down duct!). Conjunctival abrasions stain yellow-orange, corneal ulcers stain bright green. Avoid bacterial contamination. May be irritant (consider use of topical anaesthetic).

c) Skin Preparations:

i) Disinfectants and Antiseptics:

Chlorhexidine Gluconate: GSL
 Hibiscrub/ Hibitane [*Coopers*]

Indications: Topical antiseptic / germicide. Disinfection of wounds, burns, surgical scrub

Forms: Perfumed red lathering solution (5%) or 5% alcoholic solution

Use: On broken skin (not alcoholic solution) dilute 1:100

Notes: Do not mix with other disinfectants.

Hexetidine: GSL
 Hexocil [*Parke Davis*]

Indications: Specific and non-specific dermatoses complicated by bacterial infection (eg Dermatophilosis, Staph pyoderma). Also dermatomycoses. Routine coat care.

Forms: Orange soapy solution (0.5%) for external application only. 125 ml and 2.25 l bottles

Use: Topical shampoo. May be left on skin for prolonged periods without harmful effect (useful for ringworm).

Notes: Do not use in and around eyes. Do not use soap at same time.
Occasional skin sensitivity - rinse off immediately.

Povidone Iodine: GSL
 Pevidine Antiseptic Solution/Gel/Medicated Wash/Surgical Scrub [*BKVet*],

Indications: Broad spectrum antibacterial effect with some antifungal, antiprotozoal and anti virus effects. Wound disinfection, endometritis, surgical preparation, Obstetric manipulation. Routine skin care.

Forms: Antiseptic solution - non lathering 1% available iodine
    Gel - red-brown gel with 1% available iodine
    Medicated wash- lathering solution (0.75% available iodine)
    Surgical scrub- lathering solution (0.75% available iodine)

Notes:Do not mix with other antiseptics, soap or detergents. Prolonged action. Colour fades when action lost.

ii) Parasiticides (page)

iii) Astringents

Malic Acid: P
Dermisol Solution/Cream (with acetyl salicylic acid) [*Smith Kline Beecham*]

Indications:Debriding and cleansing agent for skin wounds, particularly when necrotic tissue is present (encourages sloughing). Cleansing fresh wounds. Encourages wound healing. Mildly antibacterial.

Forms: Solution 2.25% 100ml, 350 ml plastic squeeze bottles with sealed top. 30 g and 100 g tubes of cream.

Dose: pnr.

Notes: Avoid eye contact. Do not mix with other agents.

iv) Poultices

Animalintex: GSL
Complete Poultice Dressing [*Robinson Healthcare*]

Indications: Poulticing of infected/inflamed foci in feet and skin. Encouraging pus drainage.

Forms: Single pieces of impregnated bandage with plastic backing sheet.

Dose: Change pnr

Notes: Useful for softening foot more than anything!

Kaolin: GSL
Indications: Poulticing skin and foot infections.

Forms: Paste for topical application.

Dose: Change pnr

Notes: Messy and smelly!

v) <u>Casting Materials</u>

<u>Plaster of Paris</u>
Gypsona

<u>Indications</u>: Immobilisation of fractures, granulating wounds etc

<u>Forms</u>: Impregnated bandages in dehydrated foil wrapped packs (various sizes)

<u>Notes</u>: Slow setting (warmth if normal). Useless if hydrated/packet burst etc. Heavy and liable to cracking, softening if allowed to get wet. Protective waterproofing is available as emulsion applied after drying (*Plasterlac*).

<u>Synthetic polyacrilic</u>
Scotchcast [*3M*]

<u>Indications</u>: Immobilisation of fractures, dislocations and granulating wounds etc.

<u>Forms</u>: Individual wrapped bandages to be soaked in water immediately prior to use

<u>Notes</u>: Use proprietary adhesive sponge with appropriate cut out portions over pressure points and round top of cast.
Wear gloves as compound very sticky and persistent!

d) Joint preparations:

<u>Polysulphated glycosaminoglycan (PSGAG)</u>:   POM
    Adequan [*Panpharma*]

<u>Indications</u>: Treatment of lameness due to degenerative (aseptic/closed) joint disease of traumatic origin.

<u>Forms</u>: Aqueous solution for intra-articular injection 250 mg/ml in 1 ml single dose ampoules. 100mg/ml in 5 ml ampoules for single im injection.

<u>Dose</u>: Single ampoule (250 mg) (1ml) injected into affected joint weekly for 5 weeks. Im injection 5 ml (100mg/ml) every 3 - 4 days for 7 injections.

<u>Notes</u>: **Ensure asepsis!** DO NOT inject into infected joints, or non-infected joints with significant soft tissue inflammation. Do not use if renal or hepatic disease. May be transient swelling. If severe reaction discontinue.

<u>Sodium Hyaluronate</u>:   POM
    Equron [*Duphar*]#, Hylartil vet [*Fisons/Pharmacia*]*, Hyalovet 20 [*C-Vet*]*

<u>Indications</u>: Intra-articular treatment of joint disease (only **closed** trauma and degenerative joint disease)

<u>Forms</u>:
    # Single dose preloaded syringes containing 2 ml (5 mg/ml)(intra-articular)
    * Purified hyaluronic acid 10 mg/ml in 2 ml preloaded syringes.

<u>Dose</u>:Intra-articular injection (2ml for small joints/ 4 ml for larger joints)
    Repeat doses at 1 - 4 weeks pnr.

<u>Notes</u>: **Ensure aseptic injection.** Transient swelling may be produced. No more than 2 joints to be treated at any one time. Horse should receive controlled exercise for 7 - 10 days after injection. Intramuscular route possible but wasteful. If no change - consider diagnosis! Useful as anterior chamber dilating agent in eye surgery!

e) Antidotes and antitoxins:

Dimercaprol:

Indications: Heavy metal intoxication (As, Pb, Hg).

Forms: Injection in oil.

Dose: 3 - 5 mg/kg q 6h IM

Notes: May be used at low dosages simultaneously with CaEDTA.

Sodium Calcium Edetate: POM
Sodium Calcium Edetate 25% [*Animalcare*]

Indications: Lead intoxication.

Forms: 200 mg/ml injection.

Dose: 110 mg/kg q 24h IV diluted 1:4 from concentrate 25%. Repeated injections every 48 - 72 hours for 3 doses.

Notes: Lower doses may be indicated when other antidotes are given simultaneously.

Sodium Nitrite:

Indications: Cyanide poisoning.

Forms: 30 mg/ml injection.

Dose: 10 - 20 mg/kg IV.

Notes: Most effective when used with sodium thiosulphate.

Sodium thiosulphate:

Indications: Cyanide poisoning.

Forms: 250 mg/ml injection

Dose: 250 - 500 mg/kg IV, may be repeated.

Notes: Seldom in time!

f) Suture Materials

NAME	Material	Character*	Gauges (metric)	T$_{1/2}$ (days)	Colour
-	catgut	AB NAT	2-5	5-7	beige
-	chromic catgut	AB NAT	1-8	10-12	beige
Vicryl	polyglactin 910	AB SYN BR#	0.4-5	14	purple
Dexon	polyglyc acid	AB SYN BR ~	0.7-5	10	green
PDS	polydioxanone	AB SYN MONO	0.5-5	35	blue
Supramid	polyamide(nyl)	NA SYN SHTH	0.5-8	n/a	white
Vetafil	polyamide	NA SYN SHTH	1.5-7	n/a	white
Ethibond	polyester	NA SYN BR #	O.5-7	n/a	green
Ethilon	polyamide(nyl)	NA SYN MONO	0.7-5	n/a	blue
Prolene	polypropylene	NA SYN MONO	1-4	n/a	blue
Mersilk	silk	NA NAT BR	0.2-5	n/a	black
-	linen	NA NAT BR	2-5	n/a	white
Michels clips	st. steel	NA SYN	-	n/a	metallic

*
AB = absorbable	BR = Braided	# = Coated
NA = non absorbable	SHTH = Sheathed	~ = some types coated
SYN = synthetic	MONO = Monofilament	
NAT = natural	(nyl) = Nylon	

Drugs contraindicated in the Horse

Amoxycillin: Severe local reactions. Specific IV form may be safe.

Lincomycin: Diarrhoea, Colitis, Laminitis, Shock

Oxytetracycline: Fungal overgrowth diarrhoea

Amitraz: severe CNS effects, Shock

Cortisone: (see notes), Laminitis

Trimethoprim-sulphur with Detomidine: serious cardiac arrythmia

Tylosin

NOTES

NOTES

NOTES

NOTES

APPENDICES

APPENDIX 1

BODY WEIGHT ESTIMATION:

Formula for estimation of body weight:

$$\text{WEIGHT (KG)} = \frac{\text{Length(cms)} \quad x \quad \text{Girth(cms)}^2}{12000}$$

$$\text{WEIGHT (LB)} = \frac{\text{Length(ins)} \quad x \quad \text{Girth(ins)}^2}{300}$$

Where :   length = point of shoulder to point of buttock
girth = thoracic girth behind point of elbow

Note: where calculator is available a more accurate weight can be obtained from the following formula:

$$\text{Wt (KG)} = \frac{\text{Length(cms)}^{0.97} \quad x \quad \text{Girth(cms)}^{1.78}}{3011}$$

where: length = point of elbow to point of buttock
girth = umbilical girth
(Jones and others, 1990)

APENDIX 2:

METRIC - IMPERIAL CONVERSION CHARTS

Weight
1 pound = 454 g
2.2 lb = 1000g = 1kg
1 grain = 65 g
1 oz   = 28 g
1 grain(gr) = 65 mg

Volume/Capacity
1 gallon = 3.8 l
1 quart(2pt)= 950 ml
1 litre = 1.76 pints

Temperature

$9x(°C) = (5 \times °F)-160$

$°C = (°F-32)x\ 0.555$

Length

1 inch = 2.54 cm
1 foot = 30.48 cm
1 yard = 0.914 m

MOLECULAR WEIGHTS

COMPOUND	MOLECULAR WEIGHT	EQUIVALENT WEIGHT
Sodium Chloride	58	58
Sodium Bicarbonate	84	84
Sodium Acetate (anhydrous)	82	82
Sodium Acetate (trihydrate)	136	136
Sodium Lactate	112	112
Potassium Chloride	75	75
Calcium Gluconate	430	215
Calcium Lactate (anhydrous)	218	114
Calcium Chloride	111	56.5
Magnesium Sulphate ($5H_2O$)	246	123

Molecular weights important in preparation of parenteral fluid therapy solutions.
1 milliequivalent is 0.001 of the equivalent weight in one litre of water

164

APPENDIX 3:

SI- OLD UNIT CONVERSION FACTORS
(SOME HELP FOR OLD FRIENDS!)

NOTE: i) TRY TO AVOID USING THE "OLD" UNITS!
ii) Have you tried the SI units? They really are BETTER!

Conversion Factors (old and SI units):

	SI units	Old units	old->SI conversion
Erythrocyte Count (RBC)	$x10^{12}/L$	$x10^6/mm^3$	$x\ 10^6$
Haematocrit (PCV)	L/L	%	x 0.01
Haemoglobin (Hb)	g/L	g/100ml	x 10
Mean cell Vol(MCV)	fl	μm^3	no change
Mean cell Hb conc(MCHC)	g/l	%	no change
Mean corp Hb (MCH)	pg	pg	no change
Leucocyte Count (WBC)	$x10^9/L$	$x10^3/mm^3$	$x\ 10^6$
Total serum protein (TSP)	g/L	g/100ml	x 10
Albumin (Alb)	g/L	g/100ml	x 10
Globulin (Glob)	g/L	g/100ml	x 10
Bilirubin (Bilir)	$\mu mol/L$	mg/100ml	x 17.1
Cholesterol (Chol)	mmol/L	mg/100ml	x 0.026
Creatinine (Creat)	$\mu mol/L$	mg/100ml	x 88.4
Glucose (Gluc)	mmol/L	g/100ml	x 0.056
Urea (BUN)*	mmol/L	mg/100ml	. x 0.167
Calcium (Ca)	mmol/L	mg/100ml	x 0.25
Inorganic phosphate (PO₄)	mmol/L	mg/100ml	x 0.323
Sodium (Na)	mmol/L	mEq/l	no change
Potassium (K)	mmol/L	mEq/L	no change
Magnesium (Mg)	mmol/L	mEq/L	no change
Chloride (Cl)	mmol/L	mEq/L	no change
Enzymes (all)	iu/L	mU/ml	no change
T_3 / T_4 (T3 / T4)	nmol/l	ng/ml	x 1.29

* to convert BUN to urea multiply by 2.14

AGEING OF HORSES

Table of tooth eruption times:

Tooth	Milk	Permanent
Central	0-1 wk	$2^1/_2$ y
Lateral	2-4 wk	$3^1/_2$ y
Corner	7-9 mth	$4^1/_2$ y
Premolar2	2-8 wk	$2^1/_2$ y
Premolar3	2-8 wk	3 y
Premolar4	2-8 wk	4 y
Molar1	n/a	1 y
Molar2	n/a	2 y
Molar3	n/a	$3^1/_2$ y

Wear Pattern of Incisor Teeth (approximate):

	Age (years) for LOWER INCISORS		
	CENTRAL	LATERAL	CORNER
	5-6	6-7	7-9
	8-9	9-10	10-12
	11-12	12-14	13-15
	13-15	15-18	16-20
	>20	>25	>25

Infundibulum
Enamel
Dentine
Cement
Pulp Cavity

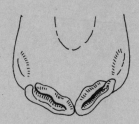

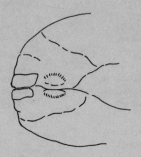

1 WEEK

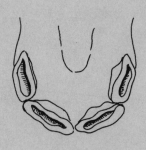

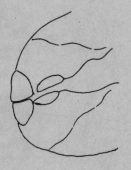

1 MONTH

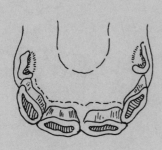

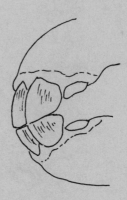

1 YEAR

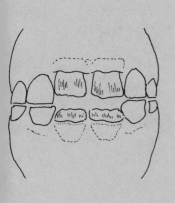

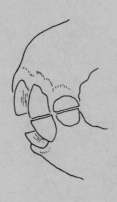

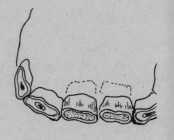

3 YEARS

168

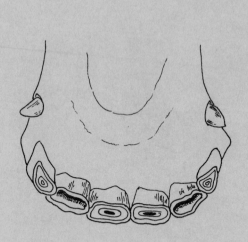
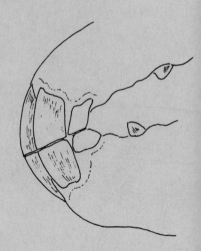

4 YEARS

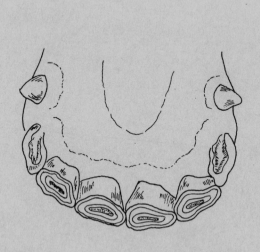
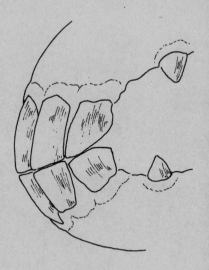

5 YEARS

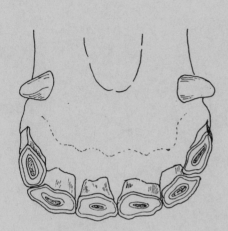 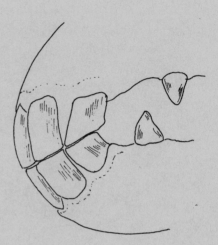

6 YEARS

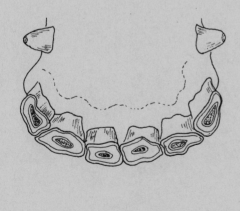 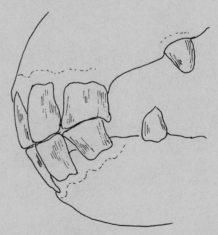

7 YEARS

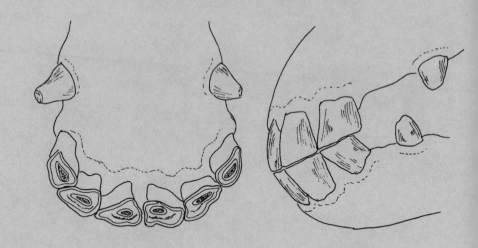

8 YEARS

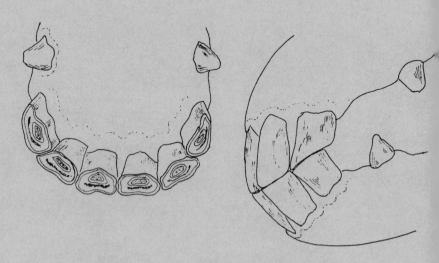

9 YEARS

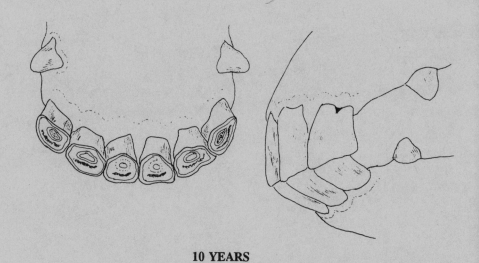

10 YEARS

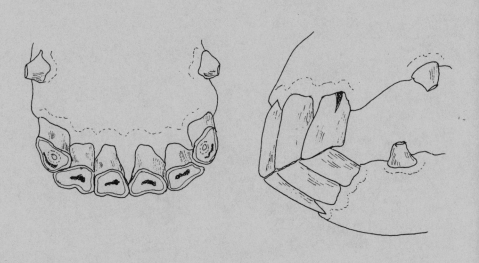

13 YEARS

172

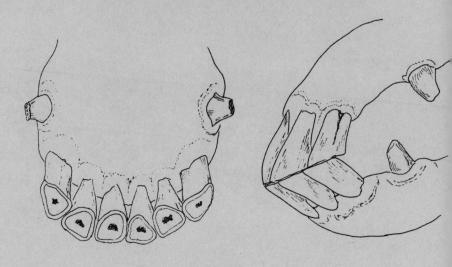

15 YEARS

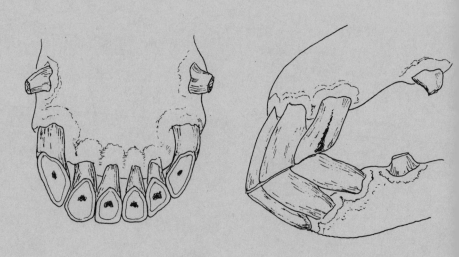

> 20 YEARS

APPENDIX 5

SITE FOR HUMANE DESTRUCTION OF HORSES

Note: It is not safe to employ a captive bolt weapon for destruction of horses (RCVS Emergency Measures Leaflet). May be effective in skilled hands and pithing is necessary after its use.

All persons using firearms for any purpose are required by law to hold a valid **Firearms Certificate** (Firearms Act, 1982).

All possible **precautions** must be taken to ensure that human lives are not risked when using firearms. Take particular care to clear the area behind the horse.

Shotguns and rifles are difficult to handle and use effectively (Do not shoot from a distance unless you have a suitable weapon and experience!). The **minimum acceptable calibre** of weapon is 0.32 using a heavy soft nose with a **strong** charge rating.
Do not try to use a 0.22 calibre weapon!

The **site for destruction** is the point of intersection of lines drawn from the medial canthus of the eye to the middle of the opposite ear (see diagram).

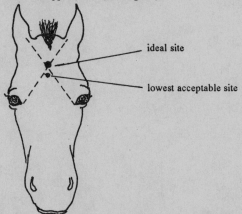

ideal site

lowest acceptable site

A useful quick method for locating ideal site is measure from the base of the forlock with two fingers width (for ponies < 14hh), three fingers width (for larger ponies and small horses - 14hh-16h) or four fingers width (over 16 hh). The muzzle of the weapon is placed just below this level in the midline. Aim down cord ie not at right angles to frontal bone (too low).

DO NOT LEAVE YOUR FINGERS THERE!

The muzzle of the pistol should be held a few millimeters away from the skull. However, in the event of uncertainty the muzzle may be rested gently on the skin.It is sometimes helpful to **blindfold or sedate (or even anaesthetise)** the horse.

IF YOU ARE UNCERTAIN OF THE METHOD THEN DO NOT SHOOT THE HORSE!

Alternative methods include: Barbiturate drugs (Always use a fast acting form first possibly with succinylcholine, rather than pentobarbitone), Aortic severance, Potassium chloride and other combinations of electrolytes and anaesthetic agents.

It is impossible to destroy a horse solely with ether, chloroform or halothane etc.

APPENDIX 5

BANDAGING TECHNIQUES FOR HORSES

A) Bandaging the foot: NOTE: bandage may "ride up" so ensure top adhesive is crossed under heels/foot.

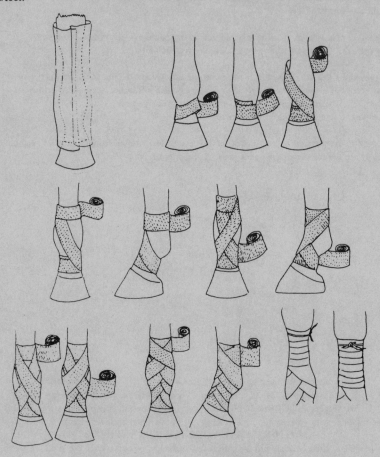

B) Bandaging the Knee and Hock:

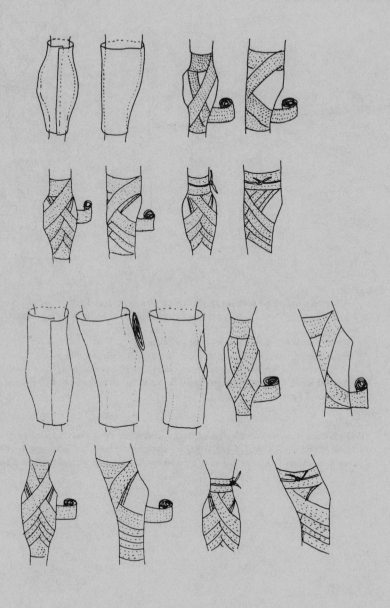

C) Robert Jones Bandage:

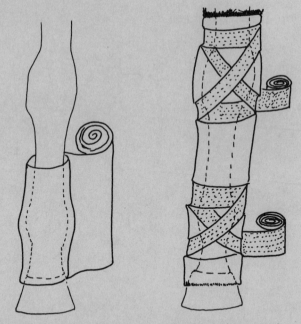

Method:

i) Cotton wool rolled onto leg to give two layers over entire length to be incorporated

ii) Conforming cotton bandage drawn firmly over entire length avoiding pressure points.

iii) Further layer of cotton wool over entire length

iv) Further bandages applied over entire length (including pressure points.

v) Successive layers of cotton wool and bandage to provide 4 - 6 layers.

The finished Robert Jones Bandage should be hard and should respond like wood to a firm flick with the finger.

NOTE: Horses with ruptured/sprained flexor tendons or suspensory apparatus or distal limb fractures MUST be <u>AXIALLY LOADED</u> ie. block under heel and splint up front of limb as high up as practicable and in any case beyond the knee. Strap leg tightly before transport.

APPENDIX 7

ROUTINE DIAGNOSTIC NERVE BLOCK SITES

Note: These sites may also be used where analgesia is required.

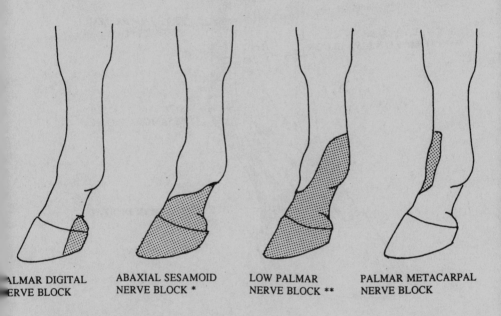

ALMAR DIGITAL
ERVE BLOCK

ABAXIAL SESAMOID
NERVE BLOCK *

LOW PALMAR
NERVE BLOCK **

PALMAR METACARPAL
NERVE BLOCK

* Palmar Nerve Block - at base of proximal sesamoid bone

** Palmar Nerve Block - just above fetlock

SKIN AREAS DESENSITISED BY DIAGNOSTIC NERVE BLOCKS

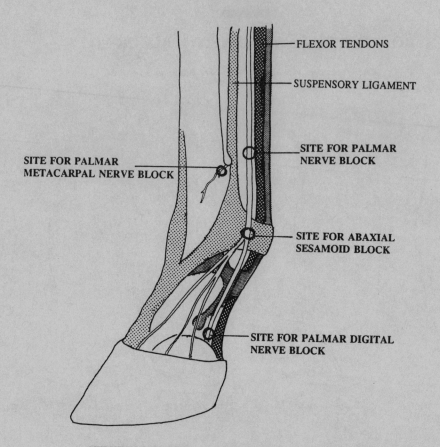

FLEXOR TENDONS

SUSPENSORY LIGAMENT

SITE FOR PALMAR
NERVE BLOCK

SITE FOR PALMAR
METACARPAL NERVE BLOCK

SITE FOR ABAXIAL
SESAMOID BLOCK

SITE FOR PALMAR DIGITAL
NERVE BLOCK

NERVE BLOCK SITES ON THE LOWER LIMB OF THE HORSE

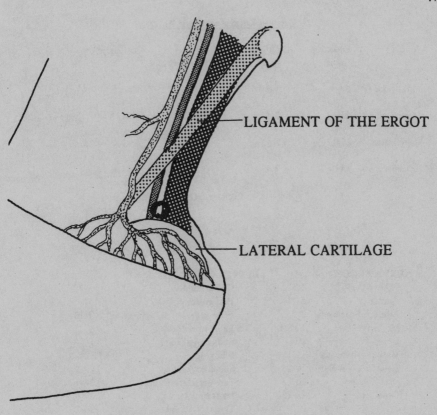

LIGAMENT OF THE ERGOT

LATERAL CARTILAGE

DETAIL OF PALMER DIGITAL BLOCK SITE

Table of Local Anaesthetic Agents:

AGENT	Onset (mins)	Duration (hrs)	Relative Potency*	Irritancy*
Lignocaine	5	1-2	1	-
Mepivicaine	11/12	2-4	1	less
Bupivicaine	11/12	2-5	2-4	less
Procaine	15	<1	0.5	-

* compared to Lignocaine Hydrochloride

Guide to volumes of Lignocaine Hydrochloride (2%) used:

a) NERVE BLOCK (ml)

Palmar Digital	1.5-2.0
Palmar	5
Palmar Metacarpal	3-5
Median	10-20
Ulnar	10
Musculocutaneous	10
Superficial Fibular	10-15
Deep Fibular	10-15
Tibial	15-25

b) INTRA-ARTICULAR (ml)

Coffin Joint	5-7
Pastern Joint	5
Fetlock Joint	7-10
Intercarpal Joint	5
Radiocarpal Joint	5
Elbow Joint	10-20
Shoulder Joint	-
Tarsometatarsal Joint	3-5
Intertarsal Joint	3
Tibiotarsal Joint	10-20
Femoropatellar Joint	30-50
Lateral Femeropatellar Joint	20-30
Hip Joint	-
Sacroiliac	-

c) BURSAL ANAESTHESIA (ml)

Navicular Bursa	5
Cunean Bursa	8

APPENDIX 8

NEONATAL ASSESSMENT AND SCORING OF FOALS

Normal birthweight of thoroughbred foals: 42-46 kg (Primipara)
48-52 kg (Multipara)

NORMAL FOAL ASSESSMENT AT BIRTH:

TIME	Temperature (°C)	Pulse (/min)	Resp Rate (/min)	Notes
0-1min	37 -37.5	70	70	Hypoxia/metab + resp acidosis
5-30min	36.8-37.0	120	50	cord rupture/shivering/righting attempts to stand/sucking reflex
30-60min	37.5-38.2	140	40	Co-ordination/standing Maternal recognition
1 - 2hr	38.0	120	35	Teat seeking, follows mare
2 - 12hr	38.0	100	35	Meconium/urine passed COLOSTRUM ESSENTIAL
12 - 48hr	38	90	30	Bonding. Closure of FO+DA NO more colostral absorbtion

BIRTH SCORE
(assessed in first 5 minutes of life)

SCORE	0	1	2
HEART RATE	Undetectable	< 60	> 60
RESPIRATORY RATE	Undetectable	Slow/Irregular	Regular > 60
MUSCLE TONE	LIMP	Flexed extremities	Sternal recumbency
NASAL RESPONSE	NIL	Grimace/Movement	Sneeze/Rejection

INTERPRETATION: Normal foals score 7-8
Moderate depression 4-6
Marked depression 1-4
DEAD 0

SEPSIS SCORING OF FOALS:

	FACTOR	4	3	2	1	0	VALUE
HISTORY	High Risk Foaling		YES			NO	
	Pre/dys- mature (Gestational days)		< 300	300-310	311-330	> 331	
HAEMATOLOGY	Neutrophils (x10⁹/l)		< 2.0	2.0-4.0	4.0-8.0	NORMAL	
	Band Neutrophils (x10⁹/l)		> 0.2	0.05-0.2		< 0.05	
	Toxic Neutrophils (x10⁹/l)	++++	+++	++	+	0	
BIOCHEMISTRY	Fibrinogen (g/l)			> 6.0	3.0-6.0	< 3.0	
	Glucose (mmol/l)			< 3.0	3.0-4.5	> 4.5	
	IgG (g/l)#	< 2.0	2.0-4.0	4.0-6.0	6.0-8.0	> 8.0	
CLINICAL SIGNS	Petechiae/Scleral injection *		+++	++	+	NIL	
	Pyrexia (°C)			> 39	38-39	NORMAL	
	Hypotonia/Coma/Depression/Convulsions			MARKED	MILD	NIL	
	Uveitis/Diarrhoea/Dyspnoea/Joint Ill /Wounds		YES			NO	

TOTAL

= Zinc Sulphate Turbidity   * NOT associated with trauma
SCORE: >11 = SEPSIS; <11 NON-SEPSIS (90% accurate)

APPENDIX 9

NOTIFIABLE DISEASES

1) AFRICAN HORSE SICKNESS (Africa, Middle East, Spain/Potugal)

2) ANTHRAX (Worldwide)

3) DOURINE (T equiperdum) (Africa, Far East, Middle East)

4) EQUINE ENCEPHALOMYELITIS (USA/Canada/South America/Asia/Japan)

5) EPIZOOTIC LYMPHANGITIS (Africa/Asia/Mediterranean)

6) EQUINE INFECTIOUS ANAEMIA (Europe/Africa/Asia)

7) GLANDERS/FARCY (Asia/Africa)

9) PARASITIC MANGE (worldwide)

10) RABIES (worldwide)

11) Contagious Equine Metritis

Note: Salmonellosis and Warble Fly not strictly notifiable in the horse but suspect cases should be reported to Local Ministry Officials (DVO).

APPENDIX 10

INVESTIGATIVE METHODS:

1) PURCHASE EXAMINATION:

a) ENSURE that you are being asked to carry it out for the PURCHASER.

b) Be aware of the proposed PURPOSE/USE. Ensure your client has seen and tried the horse. Ask if there are any points which he/she has noted and wishes you to pay particular attention to eg breeding organs or obvious problems such as scars, bony lumps etc.

c) Record details of the horse (age/colour/sex/height etc), name/address/phone number of premises (and vendor if different). Check facilities exist (darkened box/tack/suitable rider/handler/lunging facilities, exercising yard/field as appropriate). Accurate travel directions!

d) Preferably purchaser to be present with you when examination done.

e) Arrange appointment with VENDOR (ensuring horse is kept stabled overnight until you arrive). Give accurate time of arrival and arrive 10-15 minutes early!

f) On arrival: observe yard & attitude of vendor (helpful/resentful/over talkative etc!). Observe horse from distance. In presence of third party ASK vendor if there is anything he/she wants to tell you. Enquire about VICES, disease (eg lameness, coughing, colic etc) and drugs. RECORD YOUR FINDINGS IN YOUR OWN NOTEBOOK as you go along.

g) Clinical examination: Observe restraint/haltering. Record age, sex, type and colour. Full clinical examination (include dark room ophthalmoscopy/thoracic auscultation). Palpate entire body surface area! Scars eg Hobday, Laparotomy and swellings etc may be palpable but not visible! Joint manipulations. If required make approximate measurement.

h) Preliminary Trot: In hand walk + trot (straight line 30-40 metres, circles, turns, backing). Sharp turns left and right. Flexion tests (whole limb) on all four limbs. Ensure handler does not affect gait or does not try to alter the gait/behaviour etc.

i) Strenuous Exercise: Tack up. Observe at all paces under saddle or lunge (if appropriate). Listen for clarity of wind. Vary exercise extent with purpose/fitness. Ausculate heart/lungs and palpate feet and legs at end of exercise.

j) Period of Rest: IN BOX without tack etc. Observe (DO NOT LEAVE). Complete ID. Discuss (in private) with purchaser if present. Check cardiac rate/rhythm and character of horse.

k) Second trot and foot examination: Trot stright from box. Full range of flexion tests again.

It is unlikely that this examination can be completed properly in less than 1.5 - 2 hours.

l) Documentation: Complete full BVA/RCVS approved form. DO NOT USE OTHER TYPES! State findings on the form eg " was heard to cough once" etc (ALL.. no matter how small/ apparently irrelevant!). Give honest opinion! Few horses will be perfect (if they are it pays to be extra suspicious!). Remind purchasers of the WARRANTY clause on the form re: height, vices, ability, adminstration of drugs. Point out what you have not done eg radiographs, rectal examination etc. DO NOT DISCUSS YOUR FINDINGS WITH THE VENDOR.

2) <u>COLIC PROTOCOL</u>

Note: Early referral of colic cases maximises the chances of survival if surgery is indicated. Not only is the horse pleased but the owner takes a live, useful horse home. Furthermore the referring veterinary surgeon has the chance of a good nights sleep!

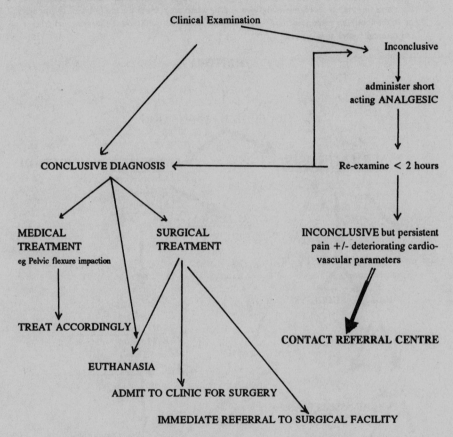

Clinical Examination

Inconclusive

administer short acting ANALGESIC

CONCLUSIVE DIAGNOSIS ← Re-examine < 2 hours

MEDICAL TREATMENT
eg Pelvic flexure impaction

SURGICAL TREATMENT

INCONCLUSIVE but persistent pain +/- deteriorating cardio-vascular parameters

TREAT ACCORDINGLY

CONTACT REFERRAL CENTRE

EUTHANASIA

ADMIT TO CLINIC FOR SURGERY

IMMEDIATE REFERRAL TO SURGICAL FACILITY

3) LAMENESS PROTOCOL

Lameness investigations should be carried out when the animal is lame, with the typical circumstances present eg. Shod/Unshod/ After rest/ After exercise etc. This is particularly applicable to referral cases. Referral centres do not appreciate having to try to identify lameness in animals receiving analgesics and/or when they are not actually lame. If you are in doubt about the management of a referral case discuss it with your colleagues and with the referral centre specialist.

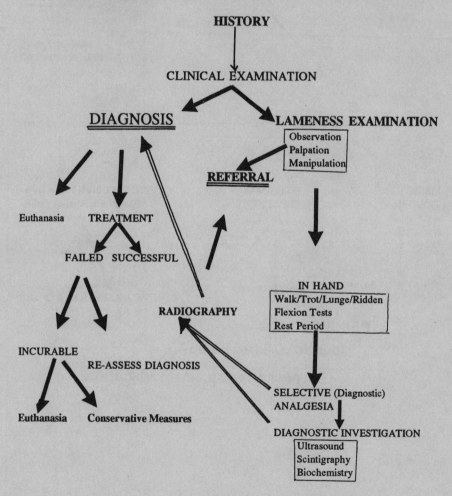

APPENDIX 11

EQUIPMENT FOR EQUINE PRACTICE:

1) <u>FIRST AID KIT</u> (for races/events etc)

    a) Euthanasia: GUN (and appropriate ammunition)*, Injectable solutions*

    b) Dressings: Melonin*, Cotton Bandage*, Cotton Wool*, Elastoplast*, Vetwrap*, Vaseline Gauze

    c) Hardware: Scissors* (Straight, Curved), Stethescope*, SUTURE KIT* (see below), BLEEDER KIT* (Clamps, Tissue Forceps,Tourniquet/Esmarch bandage), Twitch*, Tracheotomy tube*, Safety razors (Disposable)

    d) Wooden foot wedges and axial splints (gutter / 2"x2"wooden battens)

    e) Disposables: Syringes (60/20/10/5/2/1)*, Needles/Cannulae* (10 - 24), Suture materials*, Paper Towel, Sterile swabs, Sterile Gloves

    f) Drugs: Local Anaesthetics*, Butorphenol*, Detomidine*, Xylazine*, Acepromazine*, Thiopentone*, Water for Injection*, Tetanus Antiserum, Surgical Scrub,

    g) Stationery: Headed Paper*, Red/black pens*

NOTE: All items should be clearly labelled and checked regularly (at least before every event).

It is best to have the marked items (*) in a small suitcase or box which should be easily carried by 1 person and should remain with the veterinary surgeon throughout the event.

2) PRACTICE CAR "BOOT LIST":

This is not definitive and individuals may need to alter some or all of this - it may help you over the first few days in equine practice! You might even get the nurses to ensure it is all there at the start of every week! KEEP ALL EQUIPMENT (and yourself/clothing) CLEAN!

a) HARDWARE:

i) **Handling**: Twitch, Rope halter, Leading reign, Lunging reign, Chifney Bit

ii) **Farrier**: Hoof Knives (Steel/file/oilstone), Hoof Tester, Hammer, Buffer, Nail pullers, Pincers, Hoof Cutters (Diamond edged), Rasp, Apron,

iii) **Clinical**: Thermometer, Stethescope, Plexor/Pleximeter, Ophthalmoscope, Pen Torch, TORCH (rechargable from car), Stomach tubes (foal/medium/large), Funnel(s), Scissors (curved and straight), Tooth rasps (straight/angled), Gag, Stirrup pump, Parturition gown, Flutter valve, Neoinjector. RUBBISH BIN & Sharps container. Water proof marker pens/pencil. Practice stamp/pad, Headed paper. Purchase Examination Forms, RED and BLACK pens. Vaccination Certificates. LVI Stamp. GUN **(locked in a case/box fixed to floor of boot).**

iv) **Surgical**: Disposable safety razors (rechargable clippers), SUTURE PACK (sterile) [scalpel handel, scissors, forceps (rat/plain), suture needles, 2-4 prs artery forceps, needle holders, swabs, scalpel blades]. Sterile gloves. Suture materials (Catgut, nylon, vicryl). Penrose drains. Wolf teeth extractor. CASTRATION KIT (sterile: Serra emasculator, scalpel handle, two large artery forceps, blades, suture needles, suture material)

b) DISPOSABLES:

i) Roll of paper towel, Rectal gloves,

ii) Syringes (1/2/5/10/20/50 ml sizes STERILE), Needles (disposable) (22x1", 20x1", 19x1.5", 18x1.5"), IV cannulas (18/16/12/10), Vacutainer holders/needles (19x1.5")

iii) Blood Sampling tubes (EDTA/Fl-ox/Li-hep/Plain) (preferably Vacutainers - "mini" are excellent), microscope slides (in clean container-sealed) and slide carrier, bacterial/viral swabs (transport medium), Faecal and Urine pots, Sterile universals/bijous

c) DIAGNOSTICS: Fluorescein strips, Ophthaine,

d) <u>DRUGS</u>:

  i) Euthanasia Solution(s), Thiopentone (3x5g at least)

  ii) Anti-infective Agents: Penicillin (crystaline, benzathine, procaine),
  Penicillin/Streptomycin, Neomycin-Penicillin, TMS (parenteral/oral- powder+paste),
  Chloramphenicol eye ointment, Neomycin Eye Ointment,
  Pevidine scrub/solution/ointment, Surgical Spirit

  iii) Analgesics etc: Pethidine (CD), Torbugesic(CD), Buscopan, Xylazine, Thiopentone,
  Ketamine, Atropine injection (+eye drops)

  iv) Anti-inflamatories: Phenylbutazone (parenteral, oral powder/paste), Arquel, Flunixin
  (oral and parenteral)

  v) Dressings: Elastoplast, Vetwrap, Cotton Wool, Cotton Bandages, Melonin/Kaltostat.
  Poultices (Animalintex). SCOTCHCAST (carry 4 -6 rolls)/Gypsona Plaster of Paris
  Bandages (sealed tin)

  vi) Others: Calcium borogluconate (20%), Saline (1x5 l + 4-5x1l), Hartmans Solution (2 x
  5l), Liquid parafin (5l min), Duphalyte (x2), Ventipulmin, Sputolosin, WATER FOR
  INJECTION

APPENDIX 12
USEFUL ADDRESSES AND TELEPHONE NUMBERS

Animal Health Trust   0638-661-111
P O BOX 5
Newmarket
Suffolk
CB8 8JS

Beaufort Cottage Laboratories   0638-663-150
High Street
Newmarket
Suffolk
CB8 8JS

Bristol University   0934-852581
Departments of Veterinary Medicine/Surgery
Langford House
Langford, Avon
BS18 7DU

British Equine Veterinary Association
Hartham Park
Corsham
Wiltshire
SN13 0BQ

British Veterinary Asssociation   071-636-6541
7 Mansfield Street
London
W1M 0AT

University of Cambridge   0223-337600
Medicine/Surgery Division
Madingley Road
Cambridge
CB3 0ES

Central Veterinary Laboratories   09323-41111/5
Weybridge
New Haw
Surrey
KY15 3NB

University of Edinburgh   031- 445 2001
Department of Clinical Veterinary Studies
Royal (Dick) School of Veterinary Science
Summerhall, Edinburgh

University of Glasgow   041-942 2301
Department of Veterinary Medicine/Surgery
Bearsden Road
Glasgow
G61 1QH

Liverpool University   051-794-6041
Division of Equine Studies
Leahurst,
Neston South Wirral
L64 7TE

London University   O707-55486
Department of Medicine/Surgery and Obstetrics
Hawkeshead House
Hawkeshead Lane
North Mymms, Hatfield
AL9 7TA

Royal College of Veterinary Surgeons   071-235-4971/2
32 Belgrave Square
London.
SW1X 8QP

Serono Laboratories Ltd   0707-371-734
99 Bridge Road East
Welwyn Garden City
Herts., AL7 1BG

Veterinary Defence Society   0565-52737
1a Princess Street
Knutsford
WA16 6BY

National Foaling Bank   0952-811234
(FOSTERING SERVICE)
Meretown Stud
NEWPORT
Salop.

NOTES

INDEX

A...

Abaxial Sessamoid Nerve Block 177, 178
Acepromazine 42
Acetylsalicylic Acid 96
Acid-Base Balance 5
Acids, bile (normal) 4
Activated prothrombin time, blood (normal) 7
Acyclovir 144
Adrenal corticoids 93
Adrenaline 52, 63
Adrenocorticotrophin, hormone 99
                        Response Test, method for 24
Addresses 190
African Horse Sickness Vaccine 137
Ageing of horses 165
Alkaline phosphatase, blood (normal) 6
Alpha globulin (normal) 4
Alphaprostol 88
Alphoxalone/alphadolone 45
Allyl trenbolone 89
Amethocaine 146
Amitraz 156
Ammonia, blood (normal) 4
Amphoteracin B 115
Ampicillin 108
Amoxycillin 156
Anabolic Steroids 92
Anaesthetics,   euthenasia 55
                   intra-venous 45
                   local 143
                   ophthalmic 146
                   volatile/gases 44
Animalintex 151
Antacids 80
Antidotes 154
Anthelmintics 103
Antiarrhythmic drugs 60
Antibiotics 108
    Ophthalmic 144
Anticholinergics 61
Anticoagulants 124
Anticonvulsants 47
Anti-diarrhoeals 84
Antidotes 154
Antifungals 115

194

Antihistamines 69
Anti-infective Drugs 101
Antiprotozoals 117
Antisera 136
Antiseptics 150
Antitussives 70
Antiulcer Drugs 80
Appendices 161
Artificial tears 148
AST (see aspartate aminotransferase) 6, 7
Aspartate Aminotransferase, Blood (normal) 6
                              cerebrospinal fluid (normal) 7
Astringents 151
Atropine, injection 50, 61
      Ophthalmic 145

B......................................

Bandaging 174
Base Excess, blood, arterial (normal) 5
                   venous (normal) 5
Benzuldasic Acid 115
Benzene Hexachloride (gamma) 118
Beta globulin (normal) 4
Betamethasone 93
Betamethasone (Ophthalmic) 147
Bicarbonate, blood, arterial (normal) 5
              deficit (formula for) 5
              parenteral solution
              venous (normal) 5
Bile, acids (normal) 4
Bilirubin, Total (normal) 4
      Conjugated (normal) 4
Biochemical Values (normal) 4
Biopsy,   Bone Marrow, method for 22
        Liver, method for 22
Biotin 129
Bleeding Time, in vivo (normal) 7
Blood coagulation, tests (normal) 7
    modifying Drugs 123
Body weight estimation/calculation 162
Boldenone 92
Bone Marrow Biopsy, method for 22
Bone Marrow Ratio (M:E) (normal) 3
Bromhexine 71
Bromosulpthalein Clearance Test, 17

Bronchodilators 67
Bronchio-alveolar lavage, method for 21
BSP Clearance Test 17
Bupivicaine 143
Buserelin 91
Butorphenol Tartrate 39, 70

C..................................

Calcium, blood, total (normal) 4
                ionised (normal) 4
                excretion factors 23
                edetate 80
                gluconate 124
Capillary Refill Time (normal) 1
Car boot list 188
Cardiac glycosides 61
Cardiovascular Drugs 59
Casting Materials 152
Central Nervous Drugs 37
                stimulants 38
Cerebrospinal fluid (normal values) 7
Cholesterol (normal) 4
Chloramphenicol 108
                Ophthalmic 144
Chloral hydrate 42
Chlorhexidine 150
Chloride, blood (normal) 4
Cimetidine 80
Cisapride 81
Cisternal pressure (normal) 7
CK (see Creatine kinase)
Clearance Ratios, renal, creatinine (normal) 23
                                electrolytes 23
                                method for 23
Clenbuterol 67
Cloprostenol 88
Clotting Time, in vitro (normal) 7
Coagulation, Blood, tests for, (normal) 7
Codeine phosphate 70, 84
Colic protocol 185
Conversion charts (Metric-Imperial) 163
                        (old - SI units) 164
Copper, blood (normal) 4
Corticosteroids 93, 156
Cortisol, blood (normal) 4
Colloidal Solutions 132
Coumaphos 118

Creatine Kinase, blood (normal) 6
           cerebrospinal fluid (normal) 7
Creatinine, blood (normal) 4
Cromoglycate (sodium) 69
Cryptorchidism, blood values in, 13
           Test for 19
Cypermethrin 118

D.....................................

Danthrone 82
Dantrolene 49
Dentition, ageing by 165
Dembrexine 71
Destruction, humane 173
Detomidine 43, 156
Dextran 132
Dexamethasone, injection 93
           Supression Test, method for 24
Dexamethasone (Ophthalmic) 147
Diagnostic Tests, 16
Diazepam 47
Dichlorvos 103
Digoxin 61
Dimercaprol 154
Dimethylsulphoxide 96
Diminazene aceturate 117
Diphenhydramine 70
Diprenorphine, 54
Dipyrone 96
Disinfectants 150
Dinoprost promethamine 88
Dioctyl sodium sulfosuccinate 82
Diuretics 75
DMSO (see dimethylsulphoxide) 96
Dobutamine 51, 63
Dopamine 51, 63
Doxapram hydrochloride 38
Drug categorisation, 35
Duphalyte 133

E. ....

EDTA (Ophthalmic) 149
Electrocardiograph, data (normal) 27
        methods 27
Electrolytes 131
Enema (sodium phosphate) 83
Enzymes, blood (normal) 6
Eosinophil Count (normal) 3
Ephedrine Sulphate 51
Equipment lists 187
Erythrocyte count, blood (normal) 3
        cerebrospinal fluid (normal) 7
        peritoneal fluid (normal) 8
Erythromycin 109
Epinephrine 52, 63
Epsom salt (see Magnesium Sulphate) 82
Equine Herpes(1) Vaccine 137
Equine Infleuenza Vaccine 138
Etamphiline camsylate 67
Etorphine Hydrochloride 39
Euthanasia Methods 173
        solutions 55
Eye **Preparations** 144
Excretion factors, calcium (normal) 23
        Phosphate (normal) 23

F. ....

Fenbantel 104
Fenbendazole 103
Fibrinogen (normal) 4
First Aid Kit 187
Flunixin meglumine 97
Flumethasone 94
Fluorescein (Ophthalmic) 149
Folate, blood (normal) 4
Furosemide 75

G...........................

Gastro-intestinal Drugs 79
γGT (see Gamma glutamyl transpeptidase)
Gamma BHC 118
Gamma globulin (normal) 4
    glutamyl transpeptidase, blood (normal) 6
Gelatin Solutions 132
Gelofusin 132
Gentamycin 110
        Ophthalmic 144
GGE 49
Glaubers salt 83
GLDH (see Glutamate dehydrogenase)
Glucose, Absorbtion Test 17
        Blood (normal) 4
        Cerebrospinal fluid (normal) 7
Glutamate dehydrogenase, blood (normal) 6
Glutathione peroxidase, blood (normal) 6
Glyceryl guaicolate 49
Glycopyrolate 61
GnRH (see Buserelin) 92
Griseofulvin 115
GSHPx (see Glutathione peroxidase)

H...........................

Haemacell 132
Haematinics 127
Haematocrit (normal) 3
Haematology (normal values) 3
Haemoglobin (normal) 3
Halothane 44
Haloxon 104
Hartmans Solution 131
Heparin sodium 124
Herpes Virus Vaccine 137
Hexetidine 150
Homatropine (Ophthalmic) 145
Hormones, blood, female (normal) 11
            male (normal) 13
        drugs 87
Human Chorionic Gonadotrophin 90
Humane destruction 173
Hyoscine 81
Hydrocortisone (Ophthalmic) 147
Hydrochlorothiazide 75
Hyaluronate 153

I...........................

Imidocarb 117
Influenza Vaccine 138
Inorganic phosphate, blood (normal) 4
Insulin,   blood (normal) 4
         injection 99
Intestinal sedatives 81
Intestinal stimulants 81
Iron, blood (normal) 4
         binding capacity (normal) 4
Isofluorane 44
Isopyrin 97
Isoprenaline 52
Isotonic saline
Isoxuprine 62
Isoxuridine (see acyclovir) 144
Ivermectin 104

J...........................

Jockey Club Rules (vaccination)   106
Joint preparations 153

K...........................

Kaolin 151
Kanamycin 110
Ketamine 45

L...........................
Lactate, blood (normal) 4
         dehydrogenase, blood (normal) 6
                  isoenzymes (normal) 6
                  cerebrospinal fluid (normal) 7
Lactated Ringers Solution 131
Lameness protocol 186
Laxatives 82

Leucocyte Count, blood (normal) 3
        cerebrospinal fluid (normal) 7
        peritoneal fluid (normal) 8
        synovial fluid (normal) 8
Leuteinising Hormone 90
Levamisole 105
LH (HCG) 90
Lincomycin 156
Lindane 119
Lignocaine 143
Liquid parrafin 82
Local Anaesthetics 143
    Table of amounts 180
    Realtive strengths 180
    Relative Potency 180
    Relative Duration 180
Lymphocyte Count (normal) 3

M.......................................

Magnesium, blood (normal) 4
        sulphate 82
Malic Acid 151
Malonic Acid/Oxalic Acid 126
Mannitol 76
MCV (normal) 3
MCHC (normal) 3
Mean Cell Volume (normal) 3
Mean Cell Haemoglobin Concentration (normal) 3
Mebendazole 105
Meclofenamic acid 97
Menadione 126
Metacarpal Nerve Block 177, 178
Metamizole 81
Methohexitone 46
Mepivicaine 143
Methadone 40
Methindizate 40
Methionine 129
Methylprednisolone 94
Metriphonate 105
Metronidazole 114, 117
Miconazole 116
Midazolam 47
Midriatics 145
Mineral Oil (Liquid parrafin) 82
Miotics 146
Molecular weights 163

Monocyte Count (normal) 3
Monosulfiram 119
Morphine SO, 40
Mucolytics 71
Muscle relaxants 49

N.............................

Naloxone 54
Naproxon 98
Natamycin 116
Neomycin 110
        Ophthalmic 144
Neostigmine 50
Neonatal assessment /scoring 181, 182
Nerve block sites 177
Neutrophil Count (normal) 3
Nitrous oxide 44
Nitrofurantoin 111
Non-Steroidals 96
Noradrenaline 52
Notifiable diseases 183

O.............................

Oestradiol benzoate 89
Oestrone, conjugated, total (normal) 11
Oestrous cycle 11
Opiate Anatagonists 54
Oxfendazole 106
Oxibendazole 106
Oxybuprocaine 146
Oxytetracycline 156
Oxytocin 92

P...................................

Palmar Digital Nerve Block 177, 178, 179
Palmar Metacarpal Nerve Block 177, 178
Pandeys Test, cerebrospinal fluid (normal) 7
Paracentesis, abdominus 20
           thoracis 20
Parrafin, liquid 82
Parasiticides 118
Parasympatholytics 50
Parasympathomimetics 50
Parathormone, blood (normal) 4
Parenteral Solutions 131, 132, 133
Penicillin 111
Pentobarbitone 47, 55
Pentobarbitone (Euthenasia) 55
Pethidine 41
pH, blood, arterial (normal) 5
        cerebrospinal fluid (normal) 7
        semen (normal) 13
        urine (normal) 9
        venous (normal) 5
pCO_2, blood, arterial (normal) 5
        venous (normal) 5
        urine (normal) 9
Phenylephrine, injection 53
        Ophthalmic
Phenylbutazone 98
        Ophthalmic 147
Phenylephrine (Ophthalmic) 145
Phenytoin 48
Phosphatase, alkaline, blood (normal) 6
        intestinal, blood (normal) 6
Phosphate, blood, inorganic (normal) 4
        excretion factors 23
Physostigmine (Ophthalmic)
Phytomenadione (Vitamin K1) 126
Piperazine 106
Pilocarpine (Ophthalmic) 146
Pituitary hormones 92
Plaster of Paris 152
Platelet Count (normal) 3
PMSG 90
Polyacrilic (synthetic), casting 152
Polysulphated G-aminoglycan 153
Posterior Pituitary Hormones 92
Potassium,   blood (normal) 4
        red cell (normal) 4

Potentiated sulphonamide 113
Poultices 151
Povidone Iodine 150
Praziquantel 106
Prednisolone 94
Pregnant Mare Serum Gonadotrophin (PMSG) 90
Prescription, abbreviations 34
          writing advice 34
Primidone 48
Progesterone, blood, female (normal) 11
          injection/implant 91
Propanolol 53, 60
Propofol 46
Prostaglandins 88
Protamine sulphate 124
Protein,   total, blood (normal) 4
        albumin (normal) 4
        globulin (normal) 4
        fibrinogen (normal 4
           cerebrospinal fluid (normal) 7
           peritoneal fluid (normal) 8
           synovial fluid (normal) 8
Prothrombin Time, blood (normal) 7
Proxymetacaine 146
Pulse Rate (normal) 1
Purchase examination 184
Pyrantel 107

Q..

Quinalbarbitone Sodium 55
Quinidine Sulphate 60

R...

Ranitidine 80
Refractive Index, Cerebrospinal fluid (normal) 7
Reproductive Data, female (normal) 11
          male (normal) 13
Respiratory Drugs 65
Respiratory Rate (normal) 1
Rifampicin 112
Ringers Lactate 131

S....................................

Saline,   dextrose 131
            hypertonic 131
            isotonic 131
Sample Collection 2
Semen, characteristics (normal) 13
            pH (normal) 13
            volume (normal) 13
Sepsis scoring of foals 183
Scotchcast 152
SDH (see Sorbitol dehydrogenase)
Sedatives and Tranquilisers 42
Selenium (injection) (see Vitamine E) 130
Sex hormones, blood, female (normal) 11
                        male (normal) 13
                        steroids 89
Shock Treatments 63
SI Conversion factors 164
Sodium,   blood (normal) 4
            Calcium edetate 154
            chromoglycate 69
            gluconate 124
            hyaluronate 153
            nitrite 154
            phosphate (enema) 83
            thiosulphite 154
            Sulphanilate Clearance Test 18
            sulphate 83
Sorbitol dehydrogenase, blood (normal) 6
Starch Solutions 132
Streptomycin 112
Sucralfate 80
Sulphonamides 113
Suture materials 155
Suxamethonium 49
Sympatholytics 53
Sympathomimetics 51
Synovial Fluid (normal values) 8

T..

Tears, artificial) 148
Theophyline 68
Thiamine hydrochloride (Vitamin B1) 128
Thiopentone Sodium 46
Temperature, Rectal (normal) 1
Testosterone, blood, female (granulosa cell tumour) 11
             male (normal) 13
                (false rig) 13
                (rig) 13
        injection 90
Tetanus antiserum 139
Tetanus toxoid 139
Thiabendazole 107
Thrombocyte Count (normal) 3
Thyroid Hormones, blood (normal) 4
Thyroid Stimulation Test, method for 24
Thyrotropin, 24
Topical Anaesthetics 146
Tracheal Aspiration, method for 21
Tranquilisers/sedatives 42
Trenbolone (see Allyl trenbolone) 89
Triamcinolone 95
Triglycerides, blood (normal) 4
Trimethoprim sulphonamide 113, 156
Tripelenamine 69
Tropicamide (Ophthalmic) 145
Tylosin 156

U..

Urea, blood 4
Urinary Tract Drugs 73
Urine, hormone concentration (normal) 11

V..

Vaccines 135
Vital Signs 1
Vitamin B$_{complex}$ 130
Vitamin B$_1$ 128
Vitamin B$_{12}$, blood (normal) 4
        injection 128
Vitamin E/Selenium 130
Vitamin K$_1$ 126
Vitamin K$_3$ 126
Vitamins 128

W......................................

Warfarin 125
Weight estimation, methods 163
White Cell Count (normal) 3

X......................................

Xylazine 43
Xylose Adbsorbtion Test 17

Z......................................

Zinc Sulphate Turbidity Test 18

NOTES

NOTES

NOTES

NOTES

NOTES

NOTES